Look Younger, Live Longer

Reverse the Aging Process in One Year
Using Eastern Traditions
and Modern Nutritional Science

BILL BODRI

Top Shape Publishing LLC
1135 Terminal Way Suite 209
Reno, NV 89502

ISBN-10: 0-9980764-2-2
ISBN-13: 978-0-9980764-2-3
Library of Congress Control Number: 2016917351

DEDICATION

To all the people who want to live longer while maintain their health and look younger. The answer lies in cultivating your Qi, or internal energy, as well as your physical body. To cultivate your internal vital energy you should follow the guidance of the eastern spiritual traditions that teach you how to cultivate your life force, and for the body you need to undergo detoxification and subscribe to a Core Nutritional Program. I hope this book helps you achieve the goals of looking younger and living longer, which are certainly achievable, and firmly sets you on the right path..

TABLE OF CONTENTS

ACKNOWLEDGMENTS

My heartfelt thanks go to Zen master Nan Huai-Chin for inspiring me to research the topic of anti-aging and for providing an overall Buddhist and Taoist framework for life extension, Li Qingyun for breaking his silence to teach the Eastern arts of anti-aging and spiritual cultivation, Art Bartunek for his many thoughtful discussions on anti-aging supplements, Dan Buettner for his research on the Blue Zones, and Marshall Adair for lending his editing talents to this book.

Chapter 1
The 250-Year-Old Man

A few years ago a book was released about the Chinese gentleman Li Qingyun, an herb gatherer said to be 250 years old. When someone reaches such a venerable age, Chinese culture usually anoints them with the title of being an "Immortal." Of course immortality cannot be achieved, but we can strive to learn how to live longer.

Is it possible to live as long as Immortal Li? No one could verify that Li Qingyun had actually lived that long, but they could verify that he was at least a centenarian. Even then, he certainly didn't look the part. What had he done so as to live so long and why was he so healthy, happy and terrific in appearance at such an advanced age? What did he know and what did he practice?

Li Qingyun gave a number of interviews near the end of his life in which he explained his basic approach to longevity. We will see upon examination that it is not much different from the traditional multi-faceted Chinese approach to anti-aging and life extension that uses natural methods. Here are Li's principles for longevity.

DIET

Immortal Li's diet was primarily vegetarian. He mainly consumed fruits, vegetables and rice, and not too much meat and fish although he said they would not cause much harm. Because he worked as an herb gatherer in the wilds, at times he did not eat cooked food but instead just ate raw dishes.

This fact might be particularly interesting for those who espouse a raw food diet today. Bernando LaPallo, author of *Age Less, Live More*, claimed that his mostly raw food diet was the reason that he was still alive at 109. Youtube videos of 70-year old raw foodist Annette Larkins also show a woman who looks many decades younger that her true age. There are many books available which espouse raw food diets because they are enzyme-rich and produce various health advantages, and I've noticed a tendency for people on these diets to look younger than others. However, this type of diet is not right for everyone; especially, as Chinese warn, if you have a "cold-type" body characterized by cold hands and feet.

One of the secrets to long living is how you eat your food. Immortal Li recommended that one should always chew one's food *slowly*, rather than gulp it down quickly since this hurts digestion. "Chew it slowly and take time to enjoy it," he taught. "This will help to preserve your stomach and spleen energy." He was adamant about eating slowly, enjoying one's meal and both generating and swallowing saliva.

As to foods to avoid eating, Li noted that Buddhism advises against eating scallions, shallots, chives, garlic and asafetida because they tend to stimulate sexual desire in people. Chinese Taoism advises against eating chives, garlic, rapeseed, scallion and coriander for similar reasons. Chinese traditional medicine also advises against stimulating foods such as onions, garlic, chives, knotgrass and mustard.

These foods, said Immortal Li, are spices that will stimulate your body and give rise to lustful thoughts. Since those who wish to cultivate long life need to accumulate and retain their vital energies - which are normally lost because of indulgence in sex after lustful thoughts (sexual desires) arise - they should abstain from them.

Many times Li had no food when he was picking herbs in the mountains, so he and his companions would have to fast or allay their hunger with the herbs they had collected, which became their meal. Li said that with practice he was eventually able to fast for months at a time without feeling any hunger, which was an ability he developed due to his internal energy cultivation. This ability to live off air and one's Qi (energy) alone is often attained by spiritual practitioners in various traditions.

Many modern researchers have proved the benefits of intermittent fasting to life extension, but Immortal Li added some additional principles that have yet to be proven by science. For instance, he said that in winter you shouldn't go hungry in the morning, but should always eat breakfast; and in summer you shouldn't eat too much late at night. These are two life principles worth considering and adopting as lifestyle changes.

Immortal Li also advised that you should never eat to excess. This advice is like the typical Chinese admonition never to eat until you are full, but to always leave a bit of room in your stomach because of the health benefits this provides. This might sound like unusual advice, but it is a typical Taoist notion about naturally living in a harmonious fashion that other cultures have also adopted.

SPECIAL HERBS

Because he lived in the wilderness collecting herbs, Li Qingyun certainly tasted hundreds (and perhaps thousands) of herbs during his travels. He certainly learned of their medicinal properties since he sometimes prescribed them to villagers in need.

There are many herbs known in China for their longevity producing properties such as Ginseng and Lingzhi. Immortal Li specifically mentioned the anti-aging benefits of He Shou Wu (Chinese Knotweed, *fallopian multiflora*), Huang Jing (*Polygonatum*) and Baiji (*Bletilla striata*), which is an herb he advised to immediately eat raw after picking. He often ate Goji (Wolfberry) himself or drank its tea. Most of these herbs have been studied for their life extension properties, and the Chinese medical pharmacopeia advocates other longevity herbs as well.

Doubtless, these and other special herbs, especially the class known as "adaptogens," could be useful to those of us who wish to live longer. They should be studied by scientific researchers to discover whether they offer any true longevity effects if at all. The idea would be to add to your diet any safe and helpful longevity herbs found effective, but only in the form and frequency most useful.

BREATHING PRACTICES

A common Taoist principle for longevity is that your internal vital energy or Qi, sometimes called your life force or "internal breathing," should circulate quite freely within your body without encountering obstructions or restrictions. This requires a large amount of internal energy cultivation. Your breathing processes, namely your respiratory rate and the deepness or shallowness of your breath, are indicative of the health of your Qi and its circulation because your external and internal breathing are linked together. If your external respiration proceeds smoothly, because of a connective interrelationship it will help your vital energy to become stronger and flow smoothly as well.

Your internal Qi, or vital energy, can also pacify your external respiration if it is flowing smoothly within you. Thus the inner can affect the outer just as the outer can affect the inner. As stated, your external breathing – for better or worse - can stimulate the flow of your Qi (vital life force energy) within your body too. Good health can therefore be attained through your way of breathing because of this linkage between your breathing and your Qi life force.

All the highest or best life extension methods require longer and smoother breathing, which is indicative of and promotes the smooth flow of Qi energy within your body. Unfortunately, most people are rapid and/or shallow lung breathers and employ neither smooth nor long breaths during respiration. On the road to longevity, people need to learn meditation and breath exercise techniques such as pranayama to improve their breathing methods and thereby extend their lives through this avenue.

According to Taoist thinking, breathing problems can lead to short life spans, but with practice anyone can transform their regular breathing habits and earn longevity. They can do this by learning a style of deeper belly breathing called "Elixir Field" breathing, which is what Immortal Li recommended.

Li spoke of various gentle breathing practices he practiced daily to change his breathing and improve the circulation of Qi (vital energy) within his body. Science is entirely missing this aspect of the anti-aging discussion! That improvement of internal energy circulation is what ultimately leads to longevity and life extension.

If you want to live longer, this is the type of gentle exercise you need to do as daily practice. To do this, you first need to learn how to purify your mind and let go of all your worries and anxieties. Then you must practice this special type of lower Elixir Field breathing with effort and consistency. You must practice deep breathing into your lower abdomen along with various breath retention exercises to help open up your lung's capacity. Over time, this will definitely improve both your Qi and the Qi circulation of your body. Without that improvement to your life force, super longevity is impossible. *This is a major secret of Chinese longevity practices.*

THE SIX HEALING SOUNDS

Li explained that you should daily practice making six types of sound together with six types of breathing efforts in order to help calm your life force (vital energy) and open up the energy channels within your body. He explained that he did the following practice daily for 110 years, which helped him regulate the Qi within his body. If you follow the following rules and do the best you can with this practice (Indian culture promotes different but similar pranayama techniques) then longevity will be achieved based upon your efforts:

"The Six Qi are 1) Blowing [Chui]. 2) Exhaling [Hu]. 3) Giggling [Xi]. 4) Expelling [He]. 5) Hushing [Xu]. 6) Resting [Xi]. These are the Buddhist way of curing internal diseases. There is a chant that reads, 'Expelling breath controls the heart, blowing controls the kidneys, exhaling controls the spleen; resting controls the lungs; hushing controls the liver; and giggling controls the Triple Warmer.' Everyone who wants to know about the secrets for treating visceral diseases and longevity can listen to me to explain. Human viscera are the easiest to get sick. If not treating them right away, one would die. The Six Words of 'Chui,' 'Hu,' 'Xi,' 'He,' 'Xu,' and 'Xi' can treat all kinds of internal organ disease and cure them. If there is no disease, also use these six words to extinguish irrational thoughts and keep demons away. The method for self treatment is: every day between 11:00 a.m. and 3:00 p.m., close the eyes, sit quietly, knock teeth, swallow saliva, and read these six words softly.

"Heart disease patients should cross their hands and place them on the head, then intone *He* [pronounced 'ho,' the Expelling Breath] thirty-six times softly.

"Kidney disease patients should place their hands to surround the knees and intone *Chui* [pronounced 'chway,' Blowing Breath] thirty-six times softly.

"Liver disease patients should cross their hands and put them over the Jade Pillow [occiput], close the eyes, and intone *Xu* [pronounced 'shue,' Hushing Breath] thirty-six times softly.

"Lung disease patients should overturn their hands, place them on the back, and intone *Xi* [pronounced 'shee,' Resting breath] thirty-six times softly.

"Spleen problem patients should put their hands over the abdomen, bite their lips, and intone *Hu* [pronounced 'who,' Exhaling Breath] thirty-six times softly.

"For Triple Warmer problems [in the thoracic and abdomino-pelvic cavities], lay down, close the eyes, and intone *Xi* [pronounced 'she-hee,' Giggling Breath] thirty-six times softly.

"These are the best ways to treat visceral diseases. Only people who have done them can understand thoroughly and know the effects."[1]

These exercises, together with the fact that Immortal Li *worked hard at keeping his "lower Elixir field" (abdomen or "ocean of Qi") warm*, means he worked at cultivating the Qi of his body, which is the life force vital energy most responsible for longevity.

This is the secret to Taoist longevity techniques. It is not just about healthy eating that affects biochemistry or exercise to maintain circulation and flexibility but about cultivating the spiritual energy of your body, the life force or Qi that you are dependent upon for living but which science cannot yet identify and measure.

Immortal Li used a set of six sounds practiced every day in order to cultivate the health of his internal organs. There are variants of the "Six Healing sounds" used by many traditions in China. For instance, the traditional healing and longevity sounds are Shoo or Xuu (for the liver),

---

[1] *The Immortal: True Accounts of the 250-Year-Old Man, Li Qingyun,* Yang Sen, Stuart Alve Olson translator, (Arizona: Valley Spirit Arts, 2014).

Haww or Huhh (for the heart), Hooo (for the stomach), Sssss or Shhh or Xi (for the lungs), Chu or Chway (for the kidneys), and Shee (for the triple warmer).

The important point is to find a pacifying sound that works for you - which *connects with* the Qi energy of your organs and pacifies that energy so an organ's Qi feels smooth and lively - rather than to be phonetically correct in duplicating any of these sounds perfectly. "Works" means that when you use a particular sound for an organ you can eventually feel the energy of that organ or even the shape of that organ. You might even imagine beaming positive energy into the organ, or positive emotions like happiness or love, to fill it completely when you connect with its energy in this fashion. By "gripping" or "touching" it in this way you can cultivate its health by affecting it in a positive fashion. By reciting a sound for each organ that connects with the energy of that organ you can use that practice to cultivate health and longevity.

THE MIND

Li also reminded people that there is a linkage between one's vital energy (Qi) and one's thoughts, which is a principal tenet stressed in Tibetan Buddhism and many other spiritual traditions as well. "The breath is linked with the mind," he taught. "The mind and breath are interdependent, which means that if the breath calms down then the mind can become settled. To settle your mind in this way you have to spend a good amount of time in practicing your breathing," which means harmoniously cultivating your breath and then Qi in the way already mentioned.

By cultivating the six healing sounds and practicing lower abdominal breathing your breathing can become longer, smoother and softer just like a baby's respiratory processes. Deepness, smoothness and a long length to inhalations and exhalations are respiratory characteristics indicating that your Qi has been harmoniously cultivated in a positive fashion too. When you feel that the energy of your body feels harmonious all over, this is the best measure of whether your Qi is full and well balanced.

Mentally Immortal Li advised that one should keep a quiet heart in life and eschew excessive desires if an individual wanted to live longer. He explained that if you cultivated a calm mind then your spirit would be peaceful. Having a peaceful spirit, you would always be happy, your body would stay strong and you would keep away all sorts of diseases so that you were always healthy. A calm mind would enable you to avoid losing your Qi, and retaining your Qi is one of the cardinal principles to longevity. Therefore, learning mental peace and quiet leads to more robust Qi, better health and superior longevity.

Remember that despite the absence of any discussion in western science about Qi, cultivating your Qi (internal life force) is the hidden cause behind super longevity and anti-aging.

The idea Li put forth was that it isn't impossible to reach the way of the Chinese immortals who lived incredibly long lives, but you have to start with learning how to purify your mind and diminish harmful desires, which will in turn naturally calm your Qi. Normally these are all the beneficial results of meditation practice, which is why everyone who seeks either health or longevity should meditate. Immortal Li visited many Taoist and Buddhist temples in China during his travels and undertook the practice of quiet sitting that their teachers taught, which means he was definitely a proponent of daily meditation practice.

VIRTUE AND MERIT

There is a teaching prevalent in all of Chinese culture that in order to live a longer life a person had to practice virtuous ways, take an ethical stance on issues and perform many good deeds. Consequently an individual would then live longer due to the accumulation of virtue and merit.

Li actually demonstrated this principle in his life because despite the difficulty of his job collecting herbs in the wild he would often give away the herbs he collected to needy people for free. As he stated, "The purpose of practicing medicine is to save people. How can I take money for saving people's lives?" In other words, he refused to make money off of people's misery even though he had little money himself. This demonstrates a very high level of ethics and virtue and serves as an example we should all emulate.

Li would also play cards every now being sure to lose enough money in the process so that his opponent won enough cash for meals that day. This type of behavior - losing on purpose so as not to embarrass those in need - were clear signs of his generosity and big-heartedness.

Immortal Li said that longevity originated in the mind meaning that it starts – becoming either possible or impossible – due to our thoughts. He explained that if we do one good deed then our internal state would gain one point (improve) naturally. If we do one bad thing, however, then our Tao would fly away. This is because when we knowingly do good or bad things then it helps or damages our Qi instantly.

His explanation of the effect of good or bad deeds in life was similar to that of Yuan Liao Fan, author of *Liao Fan's Four Lessons*, who taught people that they should change their thoughts in order to change their fate and fortune for the better.

PHYSICAL EXERCISE

Like modern researchers, Immortal Li also extolled the benefits of gentle exercise saying that you have to exercise the muscles and bones of your body to experience good health. Otherwise your health would decline. There is a great benefit to exercise even in old age, which is when you must especially continue to perform movement exercises in order to stay flexible and healthy.

Stretch your body like a climbing bear, Li advised, or like a bird stretching its legs. Practicing Tai chi and other soft martial arts, or even yoga, would serve as similar ways to stretch your body gently while keeping it flexible and moving. In addition to stretching you might massage your muscles and bones to help keep your body strong.

Li learned the martial arts practice of Baguazhang, but never stressed it in his teaching. His own major exercise was simply walking and moving about, performing the ordinary affairs of the world with a quiet mind. This he practiced by gathering herbs in the wilds, living in nature and daily climbing over mountains and ridges.

CONSERVING AND ABSORBING ESSENCE

According to the traditional teachings of Taoism, the human organism is derived from or depends upon three essences called Jing, Qi and Shen. These correspond to our physical body (made of semen or Jing), internal vital energy (which is our life force or Qi), and mental thinking energies (which are called Shen or spirit). You can and must constantly replenish your inventory of these energies if you want to live long, but it gets harder to maintain them as we grow older.

As we age it becomes harder to easily replenish these energies, especially our Qi life force, and any efforts at life extension progressively encounter more difficulties. Taoism, which espouses the naturalistic way of Chinese living, teaches that to live long we must accumulate and then maintain all these three essences – Jing, Qi and Shen. This is the Taoist road of longevity.

This is why Immortal Li particularly emphasized the cultivation of breathing practices, for they help you not only regulate your Qi and bring it to a state of harmonious balance but help you replenish your energy as well. If you are seeking longevity you should strive to avoid losing too much Qi through excessive worries or strenuous exertions because according to Taoism this will shorten your life expectancy.

Just as an arrow shot into the air falls back to the ground after its force becomes exhausted, so the human body will weaken over time. It won't last long if too much of its animating Qi is lost through dissipation. This arrow analogy demonstrates the importance of maintaining the three essences of

Jing (physical energy), Qi (life force) and Shen (spirit) for as long as possible if you seek a longer life. If you lose too much energy or it experiences too severe a decline then the human body, as a living organism, cannot last long.

Li stated that you must conserve the three essences of the body, especially your Jing (normally lost through ejaculation which Chinese call "excessive sexual pleasures") and your Qi which he would not let dissipate through anger or extreme pleasures. Li Qingyun said that one should not get carried away by emotions, but should keep themselves in tune with conditions and remember to take things in stride because "today is just today" and there is no reason to worry about tomorrow.

According to Taoist principles, when you keep your mind empty of excessive meandering thoughts and practice peacefulness (which can be achieved through meditation practice) then this helps your Shen (mental energies). When you in turn cultivate your Shen or mental energies they will respond by positively affecting your Qi, or life force energy, which in turn helps to restore your Jing or physical essences. The most critical thing is not to lose Qi because if your Qi becomes weak you will more readily get sick due to lack of protective energy. Therefore, those who seek longer lives should pursue methods to harmoniously augment their Qi.

Interestingly enough, Immortal Li also mentioned that in the wilderness he would receive the essences from the sun and moon, which refers to a special exercise for absorbing their energies to supplement his own. There are various practices from both India and China for absorbing the Yin and Yang energies of the sun and moon to help augment your own energies and extend the life. The best time to practice absorbing the energies of the moon is during the three or four days around the full moon, and you can practice absorbing the energies of the sun during the dawn and dusk periods of each day. These are not practices that ordinary people typically know about, but are interesting to try.

AN IMMORTAL'S BIOGRAPHY

If you're interested in Li Qingyan's life and the Taoist road of longevity techniques you might practice according to his instructions then you can read about him in his biography, *The Immortal: True Accounts of the 250-Year-Old Man, Li Qingyun* (Valley Spirit Arts, Phoenix, 2014) and *Qigong Teachings of a Taoist Immortal (Healing Arts Press, Vermont, 2002)*, both by Stuart Alve Olson..

Chapter 2
Chinese Natural Methods
For Longevity

The majority of Immortal Li's methods for longevity encapsulate the typical Chinese Taoist approach to life extension. Surprisingly, many Taoist life extension techniques – even ones Li did not mention - have developed into major avenues of research pursued by modern science. Because the Taoist approaches are effective, some have even become the basis of modern sold-for-profit medical approaches to anti-aging.

For instance, the Taoist idea of ingesting placentas for rejuvenation has become the modern field of hormone replacement therapy. The Taoist alchemical mixing and matching of herbs and minerals to produce "drugs" has become the modern field of anti-aging supplements. The Taoist idea that inside your body are microscopic "worms" (bacteria and parasites) that can be killed through mercury, arsenic, sulfur and other toxic preparations mirrors the scientific approach of using antibiotics to kill pathogenic influences. The Taoists also championed many ideas in societal hygienics, predating more modern western efforts. The public benefits from instituting these Taoist principles in society included mass resistance to disease, fewer public deaths and in general higher standards of living.

Truly, the Chinese ancients weren't entirely kooky in trying to discover the principles of life or use their theories to create new approaches to health and well-being. If the earliest Chinese approaches to medicine, longevity and life science were all wrong then how come the Chinese were regularly cured of diseases? If their principles of health maintenance were all fallacious, despite their departure from typical western notions, then how could the Chinese have been able to survive until today?

TWO PRINCIPLES OF LONGEVITY

When we carefully examine the basic Chinese approaches to longevity we find two principles that most frequently stand out. They both focus on energy.

The first is that you should not carelessly lose your internal energies because those energies are necessary to help maintain your health and lead to long life. You can lose that energy through all sorts of excesses ranging from drinking to sexual indulgence to emotional extremes so such extremes are to be avoided.

The second principle is that since these energies decline over time there is a definite need to supplement them as necessary when we get sick or start getting older. In other words, when energies or substances decline we must supplement them in order to get back to an optimal state of balance.

Those are two of the major secrets to anti-aging!

If you refrain from losing your internal Qi energy and internal essences in the first place then your body will be better fit to resist deterioration and decline. If you also learn how to supplement declining energies and faculties you can then work to rejuvenate yourself and end up living healthier and longer.

How did the Taoists develop these two basic notions?

Surveying the skies at night, the Taoists observed the planets revolving in their regular heavenly orbits, and took this unbending regularity as symbolizing an endless process that lasts forever. They then reasoned that the human body, as a physical organism, had its faults and deficiencies but if it went along with nature then *it might also have an endless potential as demonstrated by the heavens*. This endless potential thus become their goal and aspiration.

The laws and physics governing man, they reasoned, most probably possess similar functions to those regulating earth and the heavens (the planets) that seem to last forever, but must simply take a different shape because of the human form and its life principles. The Taoists reasoned that if we could learn those laws of longevity and then apply them to our lives so they developed a constant regularity like the earth and heavens, we could create various means for well-being and life extension.

Nature is controlled by laws, and since human beings have minds that can learn these laws and understand how to control various aspects of nature, the Taoists believed humans could reach a stage where an individual could master his own life and manage it all by himself so that he was not subject to normal laws and conditions.

The Chinese Taoists reasoned that if a person learned how to tap into and cultivate the endless potential of life, which they identified as the Qi (life force) of the body rather than the physical body essence itself (Jing), they could supplement its shortcomings, transform the underlying physical body, and as a result live a much longer and healthier life than normal. They could even reverse old age, restore youth, and add many more years to longevity after being rejuvenated. It was also presumed that through this route of pursuit they might be able to create an immortal body that lasted forever, which is the basis of Taoist spiritual practice.

In their comparisons, the Chinese Taoists noticed that the longevity of heaven was similar to the incorruptibility of gold, which neither rusts nor tarnishes. It always stays the same keeping to its original nature. Chinese Taoists reasoned that if the physiological functions of the human body could be transformed through purification in such a way that they reflected the unchanging nature of gold that needed no replenishment or rejuvenation, naturally one could then live a long time.

As Zen master Nan Huai-chin put it, the Taoists considered that humans were originally capable of "cultivating a life which exists as long as Heaven and earth, and capable of attaining a longevity that compares with the sun and moon." Since mankind can manage the laws of nature, Taoists reasoned, why can mankind not learn how to harness the laws of life extension that govern the universe?

Immortal Li Qingyun explained part of the difficulty confronting us. When people become too entangled with external desires and their own emotions (anger, sorrow, joy, love, hate, etc.) they become unable to recognize the source of life (Qi) within themselves, and thus cannot cultivate it. Instead they end up losing it, and as their life force deteriorates their hopes of longevity are lost along with it. This is why life extension efforts always involve cultivating your Qi and a calm nature.

The second reason people cannot harness the laws of life extension is because they are ignorant of the principles of continuation and supplementation. Instead, they only focus on consumption in life and through excesses that result in loss only experience eventual reduction and decline. They never make use of the many roads possible for the continuance, sustenance, maintenance and increase of their life force, or Qi.

The ancient Chinese were masters of observation. When the Chinese Taoists saw the unending pattern of the movements of the earth and heavens, they eventually matched these movements with the consistent pattern of human life to derive various principles and methods for cultivating life and longevity.

Some Taoists investigated physical and mental training routines for life extension. Some engaged in physiological studies that involved the development of medicines and the various ways they replenished the body. Some studied the benefits of ritualistic prayer and ceremony as you find in ordinary religion.

It was out of these efforts that a large variety of Taoist approaches to life extension were developed, most of which involve either (1) the retention, continuance, maintenance or conservation of internal energies and substances, or (2) the replenishment of declining energies and substances through the arts of supplementation.

Therefore they advised remedies such as the use of drugs and various nutrients, dietary changes, the absorption of Qi from the environment, and the cultivation of meditation and personal spirit as well as worship and prayer. All these methods had the common aims of helping you counter deficiencies in your Qi and body (Jing) through supplementation whenever possible, and making sure that you maintained whatever you already had without loss. For instance, gentle exercise is a maintenance or continuance strategy since it ensures that you maintain physical strength and flexibility that would normally decline with age.

MODERN THINKING

Modern science, investigating both similar and dissimilar principles, has not yet confirmed the effectiveness of all the techniques invented and used by the ancient Chinese Taoists, but has certainly confirmed many of the avenues they developed for life extension.

Throughout all the advocated Chinese approaches, the key to note is that an individual has to become an *active participant* in order to supplement the shortcomings of the physical body and win longevity. Individuals must *do* certain things, such as participate in certain activities or eat certain substances, to actively cultivate the Qi life force of the body and extend the human life span.

The short of it is that you cannot simply take a pill and be done with it. Living to be 120 will never be the result of an expensive supplement or medical procedure. You have to do something more that actually cultivates your internal life force and spirit. *You must take steps to cultivate your internal energy.*

To do more than swallow a pill may sound difficult to some and the thought of having to do any work at all might even frighten people who want to remain lazy but still obtain the goal of a healthy appearance and life extension. We normally want to believe the claims of scientists who speculate that we will be able to radically extend our lives and well-being with a few special medicines or pharmaceutical pills in the future. However, this is just nonsense. As we will see, entropy will always have its way along these lines unless you supplement your personal anti-aging efforts of any type with some methods from the Taoist approach. The Taoists believed you could extend your life because of human wisdom, but their approach requires a number of simultaneous activities performed with consistent diligence.

As a person interested in longevity you must cultivate your entire being and wisdom. You have to cultivate your body, energy and spirit (Jing, Qi and Shen) in a special way if you want to win this result.

CHINESE PHILOSOPHY

Chinese society is particularly permeated by a great appreciation for the science and results of longevity. Although influenced by superstition, the culture still contains extremely useful philosophies and methods that can help you prolong your life and well-being. The Chinese ideas are simple and easy to apply, otherwise they wouldn't work because people wouldn't be able to follow them.

One of the core ideas of Chinese longevity science is that you must practice meditation. Meditation – the witnessing of your thoughts without becoming entangled or hooked to them – allows your vital energy (Qi) inside to arise and then, because it is free of any entanglement with thoughts, it can start opening up your Qi energy channels. These are the pathways through which your life force flows in your body. Basically the energy in your body flows everywhere, so we are not talking about just a few discrete linear pathways in critical locations, like acupuncture meridians, but an energy matrix that encompasses every cell and atom of your body, in effect creating an independent body double of subtle energy. This is an energy matrix that must be regularly refreshed for life to continue and meditation can help do so. When you meditate your life force arises and, detached from thoughts, can start to freely flow through and refresh all these pathways.

The major Qi channels within the body are called meridians or nadis, and we figuratively say there are 72,000 of them simply to indicate that they are uncountable and pass through absolutely everything - every micro-millimeter of your muscles, bones, lymph, nerves and so on. Instead of thinking of them as lines, think of them as the energy bonds between all your atoms. The Chinese way to open up all these pathways is not one of force but of silence. When you practice the silence of meditation your Qi will arise and open these pathways naturally.

Calming your mind by letting go of thoughts allows positive (Yang) energies to arise naturally inside your body. After they arise they will then perform the vital function of opening up your energy channels. This will produce a softening of body tissues that will then benefit through greater flexibility. There will also be a lengthening and deepening of the breathing, a greater clarity of mind (because the channels in the brain open), and better health and longevity in general.

Another core idea is that the process of transforming the human body is a gradual one. It cannot happen instantly but must be cultivated gradually over time. Simply put, the methodologies all require that you go slowly. The penetration of your muscles and flesh by the vital energy that arises due to meditation is a gradual softening and moistening process.

Another popular Chinese idea is that by going along with the flow of nature you can thereby reduce frictions in your life and achieve an obstructionless flow of your life force (Qi) that helps you live longer living. In particular, this includes operating in tune with the seasons and with celestial phenomena.

Chinese philosophy recognizes it is the nature of all things that they are impermanent and must perish. However, it also asserts that you can gather and supplement internal forces that are waning and return them to previous levels. By acting in tune with nature you can avoid many oppositional frictions that would normally lead to loss and the need for supplementation in the first place, but once any loss has occurred you need to return things as much as possible to their original levels and regular functions.

Therefore the Chinese Taoists developed various methods for increasing your Qi, improving its circulation so that it avoids frictional losses during its internal circulations, and biochemical approaches for renewing the tissues of the body itself. Many of the supplements they developed for physical rejuvenation involve botanical herbs and minerals to counter nutritional deficiencies and to serve as supplemental co-factors for biochemical processes.

Most of these basic ideas can be found in other Asian longevity teachings as well as in modern scientific avenues for health and renewal.

THE BASIC TAOIST RULES OF IMMORTALITY

The basic Taoist principles for longer life that you should know about and practice are very few. They are divided into two parts: (1) those used by Taoist Immortals for extraordinary longevity, and (2) those for just ordinary good health and longevity.

Food

First, the Taoist requirements for immortality are that you should never eat until you feel stuffed, but should stop when your stomach feels about 70-80% full. Excess food diverts your Qi energies from other physical functions when your stomach is taxed by excessive consumption that burdens digestion.

To experience super longevity, your intestines should be as clean as possible, which avoids the problem of fecal poisons becoming impacted on the intestinal walls and then being reabsorbed into the bloodstream where they will recirculate throughout your body. Having clean intestines also has a positive influence on your Qi. This requirement for super longevity usually translates into eating less, sometimes fasting and eliminating any problems of intestinal permeability, dirty intestinal coatings, intestinal blockages and constipation.

The ordinary Taoist dietary rules for longevity include a mostly vegetarian diet, avoiding overly spicy foods that promote sexual desire or injure your Qi, avoiding grains (note that modern weight loss experts consistently tell us to avoid "starchy white carbohydrates" like grains, wheat, potatoes, rice, bread and pasta), avoiding excessively cold foods and liquids (since the extreme temperature difference of cold liquids hitting the 98.6 degree stomach will weaken its lining), cooking most foods instead of eating them raw, keeping to regularity in your eating hours, eating foods according to the seasons, taking your time to eat slowly, and not drinking alcohol to excess. What you do eat must ultimately replenish your Qi, or life force, so it should be clean and light, healthy and easily digestible.

Qi

The second principle to Taoist immortality is that you must cultivate various exercises to open your Qi channels that distribute energy to your body parts so that your life force can flow freely everywhere without frictions or restrictions. All the major and minor energy channels of your body must open if you want super life extension, especially the energy pathways in the legs running down to the bottom of your feet. From the waist downwards in your body contains the most difficult energy channels to open. This is one reason that martial artists practice the horse stance position for hours in order to open up their leg channels.

You can practice various yogic asanas to stretch your muscles (and thus free the Qi channels within them of some tangles, knots and obstructions), and practice the breath retention practices of pranayama to force open your Qi channels as well. A famous Russian stretching method you might also try is to go to a decent stretch of a muscle, flex the muscle being stretched, hold your breath to increase the intensity of the flex, and then release the breath and the flex at the same time.

In the Vajrayana spiritual traditions designed to help you transform your body, you often try to open up the Qi channels in muscles by stretching them while feeling the shape of the muscles and simultaneously imagining that you change the color of their flesh throughout. You basically try to "grab" the Qi of a muscle in its entirety using thought. At the same time you might also recite a mantra along the muscle's length as if the sound was coming from within it. The Chinese schools typically use peaceful means to open the energy channels through Qi accumulation while other spiritual schools use more forceful techniques to accomplish it quickly. In all cases, the process of transformation is called a process of detoxification or purification that eliminates poisons from within the body.

Regardless of the path you choose to purify your body for greater longevity, the requirement is that you strive to improve your health by opening up your Qi channels, and there are many ways to do this. If you simply want a longer life span rather than become a "Taoist Immortal," you can certainly accomplish this through meditation and simple, gentle breathing practices.

Many are the methods you can use to help open up your Qi channels. Books and books have been written on this topic since there are the roads of yoga, martial arts, pranayama, meditation, visualization practice, mantra recitation, Nyasa practice, internal energy movements instituted by sex and more. The result common to all such techniques is usually better health, a higher quality of life and mind-body well-being along with life extension.

Most often your Qi channels will open naturally due to regular spiritual practice; they will even open somewhat when you attend regular religious devotional services in the right frame of mind. The general rule found throughout history is that most long-lived individuals (Methuselah, Nagarjuna, Peng Tsu, etc.) *have always been strongly involved with a spiritual tradition and spiritual practices.*

Whether it's Judaism, Christianity, Islam, Hinduism, Buddhism, Taoism, Sikhism, Shintoism or whatever, the common factor to super life extension is not drugs nor exercise but regular spiritual practices, and most frequently the practice of meditation which in many religions might take the form of prayer or devotion in disguise.

Balance

The next Taoist requirement for immortality (long life) is that your Qi and hormone levels reach a balanced state of fullness inside your body. An optimal balance of these factors is required for long life. In other words, you should cultivate a measure of internal harmony, equilibrium and balance if you want to live longer. Living longer will also usually require regular detoxification efforts as well as meditation practice, stretching or flexibility exercises, inner Qi work, and different types of nutritional habits.

Human hormone levels typically decline over time (testosterone, progesterone, ...), as does life force energy, which is why the Taoists have advised various remedies for maintenance and supplementation. To reach a state of fullness after something has declined you first need to refrain from further loss and then engage in proper efforts of accumulation. The accumulation and renewal of spent forces usually happens naturally over time if you simply rest through a period of non-leakage.

The largest or most destructive losses of your Jing and Qi are due to careless sexual activities characterized by excessive leakage. A woman can orgasm as frequently as she likes during sex since her body is designed to absorb energy from a man and regularly renews itself on a monthly basis. However, a man has to refrain from too much ejaculatory loss of his Jing and Qi since his body is designed differently, and readily feels depletion. The energies lost through ejaculation are exactly those that could be used to open up one's Qi channels for longevity.

In a married life, sexual activities can be regulated to produce life-prolonging effects, which are included under the Taoist school of sexual cultivation. The basic idea is to have sex without leakage (for the man) and to use the ignition of vital energies from sex to open up your Qi channels. To master this method of life extension, men have to learn how to enjoy sex without ejaculation.

Meditation

Another requirement for achieving Taoist Immortality is that you must achieve a stable level of concentration that constitutes a profound rank of meditation achievement. Meditation cultivates the vital life force of your body directly. It improves its level, its flow and its avenues of circulation.

While ordinary life extension requires the practice of meditation to open up your body's Qi channels, the super life extension feats of the Taoist Immortals requires more work. For that level of accomplishment you must practice meditation and also undertake inner energy practices to move the Qi in your body everywhere to open up more energy pathways. Nonetheless, if you start upon the road of meditation practice even without doing inner energy work (see my book *Nyasa Yoga* for such practices) you are sure to receive some of the maximum benefits possible.

Merit

Lastly, living a longer life is ultimately a manifestation of merit. To be able to win this achievement you must do lots of good deeds in life and practice virtue, morality, and ethics. For many, this is one of the most surprising of Taoist teachings, but it is a basic idea in Christianity and other religions that if you do good deeds and are a virtuous person then your virtue will be rewarded by a longer life. Taoists say that performing good deeds will extend your life span and that if you want super life extension, you need to perform many good deeds in order to earn the merit for that enjoyment.

YET HIGHER

In Chinese culture the highest standard is to raise the character of a common man up to the level of a long life Immortal, and then sage. Success requires the cultivation of your body-mind complex, namely both your body and mind, the connection between them, and your thoughts and actions. You must cultivate your body (Jing), its energy or life force (Qi), and your mental functions, consciousness or spirit (Shen).

Like Li Qingyun, you can rise up from being a common man to being a superior man through efforts at cultivation and refinement, but this will always require a higher degree of dedication and management of your life skills and efforts.

Chapter 3
Scientific Theories of Aging
And Their Logical Remedies

Western science has developed (and continues to develop) many theories on aging as to why our bodies gradually weaken and lose function over time. The theories attribute aging to "wear and tear," accumulated cellular damage, changing metabolism rates, genetic mutations, hormonal imbalances, waste accumulations, chemical changes within cells, structural shape alterations and more. Some theories assert that our body is designed to age and therefore must follow certain biological limits while others propose, like the Taoists, that any natural limits can be surpassed if they do indeed exist.

Only rarely do the scientists behind these various theories recommend any natural remedies to counter the proposed processes. In the light of what we have already learned from the Chinese Taoists, let us visit just a few of these theories and suggest some logical ways to address them.

Wear and Tear

The first aging theory of "Wear and Tear" concerns the detrimental accumulation of cellular abuse over time. It entails the idea that cells and tissues have parts that eventually wear out as time progresses and this results in aging. Deterioration naturally happens to most material things in life, and therefore most people readily understand the idea that ordinary insults, injuries and toxins in the diet and/or environment might wear down or damage cells that would then "age" and die.

The wear and tear of cells due to chance damage that accumulates over time (such as due to toxic exposures, over-working or random damage) seems to be a feature of aging, but is not the cause of aging. The natural remedy for reducing damaging onslaughts of the "Wear and Tear" theory, however, is to stop doing the stupid things that everyone knows will hurt you and age you.

You should avoid bad habits such as drinking, smoking, taking drugs and exposing yourself to chemical toxins (such as pesticides) since this definitely causes extra wear and tear on cells and sickness. To avoid wear and tear on the body, you should also avoid dangerous sports that commonly cause injuries and which might even be deadly.

In other words, if you stop doing stupid things that hurt you and also reduce your exposure to what is harmful this will reduce physical damage to your cells and you will be healthier, look younger, live better and live longer.

The remedy for this theory of aging is therefore to be more moderate in your living and avoid physical assaults to your system both internally and externally. Also, to help with the processes of cellular repair you can improve your diet so that it is more nutrient dense and devoid of harmful substances such as sugar. A sensible strategy of vitamin-mineral and herbal supplements can also help provide your cells with ample amounts of the substances necessary for internal repair processes.

A final point is that when proteins and other molecules that are no longer useful in our bodies break down, junk accumulates inside as well as outside of our cells. Therefore the more wear and tear you undergo the more important must be your elimination processes to get rid of cellular junk, and a wise strategy would be to undergo regular detoxification protocols to help remove the buildup of cellular wastes in your system.

Some health professionals believe that extra detoxification efforts are not necessary for anyone, and that any detoxification routines are therefore a "scam" because your body has the ability to detoxify itself without need of external assistance. However, the degree of toxic assaults on bodies today – because of unclean diets and countless chemicals in the environment that we absorb – is far too much for the body to handle without extra assistance. Doctors commonly joke that we need two livers today, instead of just the one we have, in order to be able to keep up with the detoxification demands placed on the body due to its exposure to countless chemicals in the diet and environment. Detoxification routines help purge the body of excessive toxins that have built up within the bones, organs and connective tissues and are a great assist to longevity. *Detox Cleanse Your Body Quickly and Completely* teaches you how to do this.

Overall the keys to countering the physical wear and tear of aging are improved nutrition (to supply the necessary nutrients that help your body rebuild and repair what's broken), better assimilation (so that you can digest and absorb what you need), and better circulation, elimination and detoxification procedures to help improve the cellular repair process.

Altered Proteins

The "Altered Protein Theory" of aging postulates that as we age the proteins in the body change shape, such as by twisting or hooking together so they can no longer do their jobs properly. As a result of these changes the cellular membranes lose their elasticity and become less pliable by so that tissues become unable to function. Body processes then start slowing down and the net result is aging.

In 1965, Dr. H. B. Bensusan proposed that the chemical process called the Maillard reaction caused long-lived proteins in the body to cross-link and become less elastic over time. This fits with a school of thought that pictures the body as a kind of low temperature oven with a very long 70-year cooking cycle; one that eventually cooks cells and destroys their proteins to create aging. Some believe that the Maillard reaction is in this way partly responsible for premature aging and degenerative disease.

You can see an example of this theory in action when you cut an apple in half. The exposed apple core eventually turns tough, yellowish and leathery because oxygen comes in contact with compounds inside the apple cells and changes their texture, which results in browning or "aging." The hardening of collagen in the body over time is yet another example of the altered protein theory.

Collagen production decreases with age, beginning in our twenties, and it progressively declines with each decade. If one were able to regenerate their body's ability to replace collagen then they would look years younger and stay younger too. Since collagen formation requires vitamin C, copper and proline, supplying highly absorbable forms of these substances (as well as lysine, glycine, zinc and N-acetyl-glucosamine) in the diet would be certain a way to reverse the clock and look much younger. Joint pains would also be reduced as well as strains and sprains due to running or jumping. Products like Jarrow Type II collagen, NeoCell Collagen 2 or NeoCell Collagen 1 & 3 can help you restore collagen levels so that joint pains and even wrinkles are eliminated. Other supplements can certainly help along these lines as well.

The cross-linking of glucose and protein through glycosylation, such as seen in diabetes and cataract formation, is another example of the altered protein theory in action. This is called the "cross-linkage theory of aging" and involves the linking together of two or more large molecules. These linked molecules end up progressively linking with yet more molecules, which then eventually impairs the functioning of cells and tissues and results in aging.

When too many cross-links form between cells in a tissue, the tissue hardens and loses its elasticity. This produces negative consequences in cellular biology. In the case of glycosylation, the unwanted binding of protein to glucose in various tissues produces compounds that interfere with normal cell functions. The proteins become so impaired that they are no longer able to perform as intended.

One strategy to address this "altered protein" process would be to break up cross-linkages by using chelating agents such as EDTA (ex. Detoxamin suppositories). These agents attach to heavy metals within the body, and cart them away so that they can be excreted. Chlorella, vitamin C, garlic and many other substances are natural chelators, but usually too weak to effectively remove heavy metals safely from the body. Rather, at times they tend to simply cart heavy metals from one location to another, thus spreading the problem. In terms of metals, for those worried about Alzheimer's disease caused by aluminum, lithium is an effective chelator for aluminum detachment and silica is an aluminum chelator as well.

Over time, the cumulative errors from the alteration of proteins changing shape and the deformation of larger physical structures (such as organs) causes an organism to vary so much from its original design that it can eventually fail to function and start to fall apart. If proteins in the body change shape as we age, the logical remedy is to reduce or eliminate the conditions that cause them to do so if the process is not purely a function of time.

For instance, the natural remedy for glycosylation is to cut down on excess sugar consumption in the diet (or hi-glycemic foods that readily turn into glucose), especially since sugar has been implicated in countless health conditions such as cancer. Limiting the sugar in your diet is a well-recognized key to longevity; of all the substances able to inflict damage on your body cells, sugar molecules are probably the worst. This is especially true of fructose since it damages the liver, creates intestinal flora imbalances and leads to insulin resistance, obesity, diabetes, heart disease and cancer. It basically speeds up the aging process so you should eliminate it as much as possible from your diet.

It is also possible to consume helpful anti-glycosylation supplements, such as the amino acid carnosine, resveratrol, alpha-lipoic acid, vitamin C and benfotiamine. Sulfurated proteins (such as in the cottage cheese and flax seed oil combination recommended by the Budwig diet) might also help to thwart any cellular membrane hardening processes, though the evidence for this approach is as yet inconclusive. Choline, lecithin, phosphatidylserine and centrophenoxine are also considered possible nutritional assists to restoring fluidity in cellular membranes.

Yet another proven way to restore the fluidity, elasticity and permeability of cellular membranes is by consuming sources of beta-sitosterol and phytosterols, which are an essential part of the "Mediterranean diet." Membrane permeability governs insulin resistance, and restoring membrane permeability with phytosterol supplements like PMCaox has helped restore the health of diabetics. This is the approach I recommend since phytosterols can also clear clogged arteries over time and eliminate prostate problems, too.

Basically, the remedy for this particular theory of aging is a better diet and nutritional supplementation.

Free Radicals

The "Free Radical" theory of aging proposes that free radicals, which are molecules having an extra electron creating a negative charge, damage the macromolecular components of cells, which then gives rise to the symptoms of aging. The idea is that free electrons react with healthy cellular molecules in a destructive way, producing accumulated damage that eventually causes cells and then organs to stop functioning.

If this theory is correct, then since your diet and lifestyle factors (smoking, alcohol consumption, etc.) are the accelerators of free radical damage this means that changing your lifestyle to avoid these factors will reduce aging. Once again you should aim for a healthier diet and better habits to counter the underpinnings of this theory of aging.

Furthermore, while your body does possess some natural antioxidants (in the form of enzymes) that help to curb the dangerous build-up of free radicals, it makes sense to support your enzyme levels through additional antioxidant supplements. This includes the key antioxidants that work with phytosterols because phytosterols help restore membrane elasticity so that these micronutrients (and others) can enter into cells. In particular, you should also supply your cells with additional levels of CoQ10 so that they have enough cellular energy to devote to repairs.

Lastly, because the simple processes of eating, drinking and breathing form free radicals due to the energy production cycles within cells, *slower living* will reduce free radical damage and thus aging. How do you accomplish slower living? Don't eat too much, breath slower and deeper, live life with less stress and haste as the Taoists have recommended and practice meditation.

Metabolism

The "Metabolic (Rate of Living)" theory of aging revolves around the idea that the greater an organism's rate of basal metabolism, the shorter the animal's life span. For instance, hummingbirds have a very fast metabolism and thus do not live as long as other animals.

We can understand this principle better if we examine the respiratory rates of animals and compare this to their normal life spans. Mice, for instance, breathe about 60-230 times per minute and have a typical life span of about 1.5-3 years. Rabbits have a respiratory rate of 30-60 breaths per minute and a typical life span of 5-6 years. Monkeys breath about 30-50 times per minute and ordinarily have a life span of 20-30 years. Humans breath about 12-16 times per minute and have a typical life span of 70-80 years. Whales breath about 3-5 times per minute and often live to be more than one hundred years old.

Maintaining accelerated breathing and heart rates not only requires more energy but accelerates aging due to the faster metabolism that increases the body's wear and tear. As a nutritional intervention you might address the implications of this theory of aging with CoQ10 that supplies cells with energy, B-vitamins that are involved with cellular energy cycles, and the mineral magnesium (in an absorbable form like magnesium orotate) that is necessary for stronger heart function. Magnesium additionally helps in reducing constipation so that wastes can be more efficiently eliminated from the body.

In Taoism you would counter this cause of aging simply by slower living, not getting too excited, and by slower, deeper breathing to lengthen and smoothen the Qi flow within your body. According to Taoist theory, deep breathing is a powerful aid to longevity and is preferred to shallow chest breathing. The Indian schools of Yoga would maintain this as well.

Are the Taoists and Indians right? Actually, modern scientists now believe that slow, deep breathing is probably the single best anti-stress medicine there is. Studies show that deep breathing into the lowest portion of your lungs hits the spot where oxygen exchange is the most efficient. Breathing in this way has been proven to lower your heart rate, decrease blood pressure, relax muscles, reduce stress and anxiety and calm the mind. Using the breath you can definitely calm both your body and mind, which is why breathing techniques are a cardinal route to anti-aging used in most cultural traditions.

Aren't the physical benefits mentioned due to deep breathing ones that can lead to longer lives? To counter the metabolic theory of aging, Taoist notions of living and breathing would certainly be the natural remedy.

Mitochondrial Decline

The "Mitochondrial Decline" theory of aging centers around the fact that the mitochondria in your cells produce ATP for your body's energy. If an organ's mitochondria fail then the organ loses energy, stops working and also fails. In fact, mitochondrial dysfunction or death are linked to Alzheimer's disease, diabetes, heart failure and virtually all the killer diseases of aging.

Mitochondrial counts decline over time as we age, so the enhancement and protection of cellular mitochondria would be an essential part of preventing and slowing this aspect of aging. The logical countering strategy is to supplement ourselves with materials that protect the mitochondria and improve their functioning in cellular energy production cycles, *or which can actually increase the number of mitochondria in the body*. This approach is basically a maintenance and supplementation strategy.

The substances that can actually do this include CoQ10 (coenzyme Q10), pyrroloquinoline quinone (PQQ), alpha lipoic acid, acetyl-l-carnitine (ALC), NADH, Malic acid, Fumaric acid, Succinic acid, D-Ribose, and various B-vitamins. In particular, PQQ increases the number of mitochondria in cells as well as their energetic efficiency so it is a great addition to the anti-aging arsenal. CoQ10 directly supplies the energy that cells need to perform their functions such as DNA repair while B-vitamins are critical to proper cell reproduction and maintenance as well.

The remedy for countering mitochondrial decline is thus a maintenance and augmentation strategy through specific dietary supplementation.

Mutation Accumulation

The "Mutation Accumulation" theory of aging recognizes the fact that DNA damage occurs continuously in the cells of living organisms and the accumulation of these errors over time gradually damages the cellular genetic code. When DNA repairs aren't performed perfectly (since the repair mechanisms deteriorate over time), flawed DNA molecules eventually accumulate causing abnormal gene expression and in some cases disease such as cancer. This faulty repair or mutation process has also been proposed as a reason why we age.

Cancer, in particular, is often caused by genetic mutations. Since diet, smoking and alcohol are responsible for about 70-90% of all cancers, improving your diet and eliminating negative lifestyle factors is a way to reduce your chances of cancer and thus live longer. Raw foods are often proposed as cancer cures since they supply raw enzymes and nutrients that help your body repair itself, as are various sugarless but nutrient-rich diets which make use of important natural ingredients (see my book *Super Cancer Fighters*).

It is true that as DNA mutations occur over time and begin to accumulate with increasing age, cells deteriorate and no longer operate properly. Mutations occur in DNA chromosomes (and in mitochondria as well) that eventually cause cellular malfunctions. It therefore makes sense to supply special nutrients in our diets, such as nucleotides (the sub-unit molecules or building blocks of RNA and DNA), to help rebuild them. Amazingly, it turns out that many foods considered "miracle cures" in the past have this common denominator that they are rich in nucleotides. Perhaps that is why they have earned such a reputation for healing and are claimed to have anti-aging properties.

To put more nucleotides in the diet, Dr. David Williams suggested that we eat the nucleotide-rich foods of Spirulina, Chlorella, Brewer's Yeast, Lentils, Beans, Oysters, Liver, Sardines, Anchovies and Mackerel. By consuming - in the most easily digested and assimilable form - the very micro-ingredients that power cellular repair processes for DNA and RNA you are going a long way to battling many of proposed causes of aging.

The practice of juicing fruits and vegetables also supplies an extremely high density of possible DNA repair nutrients in highly absorbable form, which perhaps explains why juicing diets also produce beautiful skin, miraculous cures and are said to be a remedy for aging. Fresh juicing is one of the best ways to ingest countless micronutrients that are still biochemically active. Fresh juices often contain many natural phytochemicals shown to prevent cancer, heart disease, osteoporosis, nervous system disorders, depression and more.

Consuming superfood powders are an easy alternative to the inconveniences of juicing, though this is often a lesser solution. Nonetheless "something is better than nothing," so consuming a green/red superfood powder drink every day solves the problem of deciding what fruits and vegetables to consume in order to help your body rebuild itself. Just take one scoop and mix with a liquid such as rice milk or almond milk and you are covering many nutrient bases by supplying a cornucopia of herbs, adaptogens, vitamins, minerals and other ingredients that will help feed your cells and transform your inner biological terrain. The best course of action is to do your own fresh juicing and to add these powders to the final mixture.

Nutrient dense, the superfood powders usually contain many substances such as the concentrated essences of Spirulina, Chlorella, Wheat grass, Alfalfa, Barley grass, Oat grass, Spinach, Broccoli, Parsley, Kale, Tomato, Acai Berry, Amla Berry, Acerola Berry, Camu Camu Berry, Strawberry, Raspberry, Blueberry, Cherry, Pomegranate, Cranberry, Turmeric, Cinnamon, Maca Root, Green Tea, Reishi, Shitake, Maitake, Beet Juice, and Wasabi. Packed with the healing powers of nutrition that offers the potential for cellular repair, the list of possible ingredients they might contain, in concentrated and easily absorbable form, goes on.

Two common ingredients, Spirulina and Chlorella, are single-celled algae organisms that are easily digested and absorbed, partially because when they are in powder form their particles are particularly small. Chlorella, in particular, can often help to rid your body of heavy metal accumulations and can provide many of the materials necessary for repairing faulty RNA and DNA.

Since DNA/RNA damage increases in our cells with age while repair mechanisms decline over time, remember that a possible solution to increasing numbers of cellular mutations is to consume the very foods which would be the most useful for repairing RNA and DNA. Therefore, why not consume nucleotide-rich foods such as Chlorella and Spirulina that are readily found in most super green powders?

You might also think about products such as Bragg's liquid amino acids, Barley or Wheat Grass powder, or even whey concentrate. These foods supply powerful nutrients in an easily assimilable form. Much of the work your body will need to perform for digestion is eased when you consume foods that are in the form of very small particulate pieces as these products typically supply.

In terms of the supplements that might help with genetic repair, once again CoQ10, the B-vitamins and mineral co-factors come to mind. B-vitamins are critical for proper cell reproduction and phytosterols, such as beta-sitosterol, are necessary for making cellular membranes flexible – one of the keys for countering the negative effects of aging. CoQ10, B-vitamins, minerals as well as other micronutrients and co-factors cannot get into the cell if its membrane is inflexible so I personally use anti-aging supplements like Life Assure and PMCaox (see BCN4Life.com).

Gene Theories

Various genetic theories of aging postulate that mutations, changes in gene expression and genetic error catastrophes that accumulate over time are what ultimately cause aging and death. The idea is that genetic mutations eventually occur inside cells and this gradually causes flawed molecules to accumulate. As a result, cells stop operating properly. However, since gene replication is supposed to happen in tune with a genetic clock, there might be a possibility of not just accelerating but of slowing DNA aging.

For instance, the "Hayflick limit" (the normal number of times a human cell divides until cell division stops) suggests that the life span of cells is limited. In order to stay alive cells must continually divide and replicate themselves, however, there is a limit to the number of times they can do so. Research has demonstrated that with each replication the telomeres at the ends of chromosomes (which control cell replication) shorten; and when the telomeres reach a critical length, the cells can no longer duplicate themselves.

If this is correct, and there is in fact some kind of genetic or molecular clock operating that determines cellular senescence, perhaps it is possible to slow the clock down. One solution might be to supply any nutrients that might help telomeres retain their lengths. Some scientists think that telomeres might be repaired by the introduction of relevant hormones, and at this time some people think that folate or derivatives of the herb Astragalus might somehow be helpful. Future research is sure to come up with better suggestions.

In any case, this would be pursuing a maintenance or continuance strategy through appropriate supplementation even though no one, as yet, knows what the proper supplementation should be. They do know that telomere shortening can be accelerated by unhealthy lifestyles, but little is yet known about how to reverse telomere shortening. We're not even sure this is a cure for aging either.

Another solution is to restrict calories. Scientists have observed that calorie restriction increases the life spans of humans and most animals because overfed cells divide faster and thus quickly run up against the molecular clock limits that control gene expression and aging. An additional benefit to this approach is that calorie restriction lowers insulin levels, and high insulin levels have also been shown to speed up the aging process. Intermittent fasting shows benefits along the same lines.

An easy remedy to restrict calories is the Taoist recommendation to avoid overeating and to fast on a regular schedule to avoid being overweight. Once again a modern theory of aging has a remedy in basic Taoist longevity teachings.

As to the many variations of aging theories that involve genes and their repair, a logical supplementation routine would once again revolve around the B-vitamins, CoQ10, minerals (as biochemical co-factors), membrane elasticizers (such as phytosterols like beta-sitosterol), and herbs like Curcumin that might help reset genetic switches. In mid-life the body experiences hormonal changes that turn off genetic switches, and when turned back on again these genetic mechanisms provide protection against cancer and cardiovascular disease. Full spectrum Curcumin (BCM-95) is one of the herbs that helps turn genetic switches back on and like resveratrol should be considered as part of an anti-aging protocol.

Neuroendocrine Imbalances

The "Neuroendocrine" theory of aging postulates that the body's hormonal regulatory mechanisms deteriorate over time, especially those of the hypothalamus. The hypothalamus (a walnut-sized gland in the brain) controls various processes in the body that instruct other glands to release their hormones.

As we age, the secretion of many hormones declines so their blood levels fall. Additionally, their effectiveness is also gradually reduced because cellular receptors in the body also become down-graded.

It is well-documented that age-related decline includes a variety of hormonal imbalances. Deficiencies of hormones such as progesterone, testosterone, and thyroid hormone become common as we get older while insulin, estrogen and cortisol excesses often appear. Particularly noteworthy is estrogen overload in both men and women. Estrogen imbalance is aggravated by a variety of factors including the ample presence of xenoestrogen chemicals we absorb from the environment. These look like estrogen and therefore disrupt many biochemical pathways within the body after being absorbed. They are very difficult to remove from the body without detoxification regimens.

Modern medicine recognizes that adequate, balanced levels of hormones are a foundation for coping with aging. Therefore, for those who can afford it, physicians will measure and monitor the hormone levels within your body and then prescribe hormonal "replacement therapy," a supplementation strategy, when they believe levels are too low for your optimum health. This is both expensive and very difficult to do correctly. Since natural hormones are preferred to synthetic substitutes in all cases, some people alternatively consume animal glandular products (or organ meats) in order to derive the benefits of hormonal supplementation to counteract the ills of aging.

Cortisol, the stress hormone, is in particular frequently identified as one of the chief culprits of aging. As the Taoists explained, the solution to high levels of stress - and the resulting high cortisol levels - is to take up meditation to cultivate internal peace and calmness. If you cultivate a tranquil, happy life you will look years younger, so we can rightfully say that meditation is one of the cures for aging. It will help you both look younger and feel younger.

The meditation practice of internally visualizing the glands within your body, and thereby sending Qi to those areas to help reactivate and rejuvenate them, is a powerful restorative and balancing method most commonly used in various spiritual schools. This practice, just by itself, is a useful tool for anti-aging efforts.

Waste Accumulation

The "Waste Accumulation" theory ("Membrane" theory) of aging suggests that as waste products accumulate inside cells, producing toxic conditions, the cells become less lipid, namely less watery and more solid. As age-related changes cause cellular membranes to become less permeable and less able to transfer chemicals, heat and electrical processes in and out of the cell, it becomes more difficult for cells to repair themselves and retard aging. Junk therefore accumulates inside cells, which impedes their functioning, and they die.

A visible example of this aging process would be the appearance of lipofuscin age spots on the skin, which are produced from a complex reaction that binds fats to protein. Often called the "ashes of metabolic fires," they evidence the accumulation of waste produced in cells that eventually interferes with metabolism.

Another aspect of the waste accumulation theory is acidification that extends to organs in the body instead of just cells. The idea of acidification is that too many acidic wastes eventually accumulate in the body due to a poor diet along with inefficient circulation and elimination processes. If acidic wastes – the ashes of metabolism - cannot be excreted from the body they must accumulate and become stored in the body's cells. Over decades, the accumulation of wastes that are not eliminated, discharged or nullified through normal detoxification processes then overburdens and ages the whole system.

While most toxins not removed from our body are stored in our fat cells, thus creating problems, the lipid layers of our cells also deteriorate over time when the wrong types of fats are consumed in our diets. If you consume trans-fats rather than cis-fats, the wrong fats (trans-fats) will be used as building blocks to construct cellular membranes. This weakens them because the shape of trans-fats leads to membranes that easily deteriorate. Cellular membranes composed of trans-fats therefore readily become subject to conditions such as cancer.

The first step in a naturopathic approach to waste accumulation would therefore be adhering to a cleaner diet, including replacing bad fats with good ones, so that fewer wastes and the wrong ingredients do not accumulate in our cells. Following the work of Weston Price, Sally Fallon and Mary Enig you would prefer butter, extra virgin olive oil, coconut oil, palm oil, flax seed oil, fish oil and sesame oil to trans-fats, processed vegetable oils (soy, sunflower, corn, canola, etc.) and substances like margarine in your diet.

The second step to counter cellular acidification and waste accumulation would be to practice detoxification to help clear out the body's channels of elimination, which is also a way to delay aging and work towards life extension. This not only means actions such as taking herbs to cure constipation to open the channels of elimination, but undertaking any naturopathic regimes that might help to pull poisons out of the connective tissues.

MAINTENANCE, SUPPLEMENTATION AND DETOXIFICATION STRATEGIES

As seen, there are multiple theories on aging but no clear consensus on what will work for life extension. Most of the theories focus on various types of molecular and cellular damage caused by metabolic processes gone haywire, and scientists are therefore arguing over which biochemical theories are primary versus secondary. Actually, you should consider that all these theories supply pieces to the puzzle. The question then remains, how can you slow or repair the damage of aging?

Whether we are talking about mutations in chromosomes or mitochondria, junk accumulating inside and outside of cells, damage to cellular membranes, damage to proteins, imbalances in hormones, or the acidification of tissues, one approach is obvious. That is to periodically cleanse the body of accumulated poisons, wastes and cellular debris and thereby limit their interference with metabolism and their contribution to aging. You can do this through various detoxification regimes that clean the intestines, liver, kidneys and connective tissues, which is why I wrote *Detox Cleanse Your Body Quickly and Completely.*

An additional approach is to help the body periodically repair (not completely but a lot) the various types of damage or imbalances that occur over time as we age so that we keep below the threshold level that makes conditions pathogenic.

We can do that by devoting ourselves to a very good diet and by *wisely* supplying various herbal, dietary and vitamin-mineral supplements to assist in the processes of maintenance and repair. Once again, this is the basic Taoist path of supplementation.

There are many types of cellular aging damage, but as the Taoists properly reasoned, the basis of most regeneration therapies would involve some form of supplementation to get things back to a steady state level. The proper type of supplementation – whether through food, herbs, or minerals and other special substances - can help to counter cellular damage and address some of these proposed theories of aging.

For instance, our bodies need CoQ10 to keep running, but cellular levels of CoQ10 significantly decline with age. Supplementing with CoQ10 makes sense because it would help boost our energy levels and just make us healthier. The extra supplementation also gives faltering cells the extra energy they need to detox themselves of accumulated junk that is interfering with their functions.

Resveratrol, a substance found in the grapes that make wine, penetrates your cells and works as an antioxidant to repair free radical damage. Studies have confirmed that it also has numerous benefits for anti-aging. Specifically, it triggers genes associated with slowing down aspects of the aging process, and it also enhances mitochondrial function. The herb Curcumin, such as in BCM-95, would also be useful due to similar reasons and more.

Carnosine is yet another substance with promising longevity benefits (such as inhibiting harmful glycation processes) whose supplementation has been proven to extend life spans and prevent many of the detrimental effects of aging.

The number of substances clearly proven to help with longevity is ever increasing and yet, remarkably, many people refuse to even believe that nutritional supplements can help at all while they wholeheartedly trust pharmaceuticals. This is sheer ignorance because there are many examples of supplements and dietary changes playing a key role in curing fatal diseases – and by extension adding to longevity.

Several studies of healthy people over age fifty indicate that the death rate from all causes (including cancer) can be reduced by about 50% and longevity increased an average of eleven years just by taking nutritional supplements. Vitamin C alone can add several years to the life span when taken regularly. How can one say that nutritional supplements are ineffective or useless for health and anti-aging efforts?

The western approach to longevity science and life extension is basically centered on diet, lifestyle changes and supplementation. In brief, it is oriented to biochemistry. Biochemistry, however, is only half of the equation as we saw in our study of Taoism. Western science, including modern nutritional science, does not consider the inner factor of Qi vital energy at all; and yet this is paramount for the super life extension feats of Taoist Immortals like Li Qingyun. Qi is the second half of the equation necessary for healthy anti-aging and life extension.

While diet, lifestyle changes and supplementation can delay or prevent many age-related diseases and thus help extend your longevity, as we will next see they should be combined into a larger holistic approach that also includes various forms of meditation and Qi maintenance.

Chapter 4
Shakyamuni Buddha's Ten Methods For Extraordinary Life Extension

The ancient Chinese Taoists were not the only ones concerned about the principles of health, longevity and life extension. Similar to the Chinese Taoists, nearly 2,500 years ago Shakyamuni Buddha gave a lecture on life extension in ancient India.

In this famous lecture that can be found in the *Surangama Sutra*, Shakyamuni also said that due to special practices, similar to those used by the Taoist Immortals, there were some individuals in the world who could live for hundreds or even thousands of years without dying. You usually wouldn't find them mixing with society but rather living by themselves in the forests or wilderness.

Shakyamuni said that in order to be able to achieve such dramatically long lives these individuals had to succeed at very special meditation practices, and needed also to draw help from one or more of ten major roads of assistance.

When you examine these ten roads of longevity, you will see that they are not just extremely logical but confirm both the Taoist recommendations for anti-aging as well as the findings of modern science. You can also rely upon one or more of these techniques to help you live longer, but for any of these methods to work you always must additionally practice meditation just as Immortal Li Qingyun had recommended.

The emphasis on meditation is due to the fact that only meditation practice has the power to cultivate the life force (Qi) of your body; strong and healthy Qi is the single most important requirement for an extremely long life. It is strange that few people know that. Cultivating your Qi is actually the prime requirement for successful life extension efforts. Only through meditation and other related spiritual practices can you ignite the potential energy of the life force in your body, remove the obstructions to the Qi pathways throughout your body, and allow your life-extending Qi to flow smoothly everywhere since it will then be unencumbered by pathway blockages.

Successful meditation helps the body to become softer, warmer, more pliant and more flexible because the active life force starts opening up Qi channels in muscle fibers and cellular tissues. When the Qi life force flows unencumbered through your body's tissues everywhere, that freedom from obstruction cuts down on the frictional wear and tear losses that normally accompany aging. The greater flow of life force energy also actually heals you! Meditation does not just help you produce more life energy and restore your inner Qi levels. By transforming the physical body, which is the underlying matrix that supports mental health, it can help you cultivate a more optimistic mental state. With these achievements, any other anti-aging practices you employ can then have an opportunity to produce dramatic effects.

THE SURANGAMA SUTRA

What did Shakyamuni say in the *Surangama Sutra*? He said,

"Some practitioners with unflagging resolution cultivate longevity through **eating special foods** and perfecting the **diet** of what they eat. When they have perfected this method of cultivation, they are known as earth-bound immortals.

"Some of these practitioners with unflagging resolution to cultivate longevity **ingest special grasses and medicinal herbs** to preserve their bodies and live a long life. When they have perfected this method of cultivation, they are known as flying immortals.

"Some of these practitioners with unflagging resolution **ingest special minerals and stones** to preserve their bodies and live long lives. When they have perfected this method of alchemy, they are known as roaming immortals.

"Some of these practitioners with unflagging resolution to cultivate longevity cultivate themselves by **mastering their breathing and Qi**. When they have perfected their Qi and Jing, they are known as space immortals.

"Some of these practitioners with unflagging resolution to cultivate longevity **cultivate their saliva** [the "sweet dew" salivary hormones produced at advanced meditation levels] and perfect the way of internal lubrication. When they have perfected this method, they are known as heavenly immortals.

"Some of these practitioners with unflagging resolution to cultivate longevity make themselves strong by **absorbing the energy essences of the sun and moon**. When they have perfected the inhalation of this purity, they are known as penetrating immortals.

"Some of these practitioners with unflagging resolution to cultivate longevity use **mantras and special nei-gong (internal alchemy) cultivation techniques** to preserve their bodies. When they have perfected this means of cultivation, they are known as immortals of the lesser way.

"Some of these practitioners with unflagging resolution to cultivate longevity **master mental concentration** and perfect the way of **meditation** to preserve their bodies. When they have perfected their method of mental concentration, they are known as illumination immortals.

"Some of these practitioners with unflagging resolution to cultivate longevity **cultivate through sexual union** to help preserve their bodies and live a long life. When they have perfected this method of cultivation to achieve harmonization, they are known as Jing immortals.

"Some of these practitioners with unflagging resolution to cultivate longevity cultivate the understanding of **heavenly and earthly transformations** which they apply to their bodies. When they have perfected their spiritual cultivation, they are known as immortals of the highest order."

Let's take an in-depth look at these ten basic methods that Shakyamuni mentioned and see how they match with the recommendations from Taoism and modern science.

1. Special Foods and Perfecting the Diet

The first method of special practice, said Shakyamuni, is that you could follow a diet of ingesting special foods to achieve life extension. This would be following the Taoist life extension road of proper diet and supplementation.

From today's modern nutritional science we would advise avoiding sugar-laden foods or foods that turn into glucose easily (such as the grains, rice, wheat and potatoes), foods that produce allergic reactions or sensitivities, GMO foods, bad fats rather than good fats, and junk foods which hurt your body rather than supply nutrients.

There are foods you should avoid and foods you should eat that would supply the nutrition most beneficial for health and life extension. If you avoid harmful foods and switch to an organic diet then it's quite likely you will start to look years younger.

A life extension diet would not necessarily be vegetarian but would indeed be biased toward organic fruits and vegetables where the cornucopia of intake has many different colors (since the many colors indicate many different phytonutrients). The easiest way to ensure this would be to ingest freshly squeezed juices or consume superfood green or red powders on a daily basis, possibly in conjunction with juicing, as previously explained.

Dr. David Williams also suggested that *nucleotide-rich foods* would be a useful addition to a diet since they readily supply the components necessary for RNA and DNA repair. Since many of the theories of aging have to do with chromosomal or mitochondrial errors and the need to fix both those errors and faulty repair mechanisms, flooding the diet with nucleotide foods that make repair easiest would be a wise course of action.

There are certainly foods that can also help avoid or manage conditions like cancer, heart disease, diabetes and other typical killers, but the general rule would be to eat in such a way as to attain and maintain good health. It is easy to say "eat healthy," but there are so many competing notions on what type of diet is best (raw food, no sugar, no wheat, no GMOs, etc.) that it is difficult to separate wisdom from radicalism.

Along these lines I prefer the balanced food guidelines espoused by the Price Pottenger Foundation: eat whole, fresh, unprocessed (non-GMO) natural foods; eat only foods that will spoil; eat naturally raised or wild proteins (fish, chicken, beef, etc.); eat whole (full-fat), naturally produced milk products, preferably raw milk and fermented products such as whole yoghurt, kefir, whole cheese and fresh raw sour cream; use only traditional fats and oils (butter, animal fats, extra virgin olive oil, expeller pressed sesame and flax oil, coconut oil, palm kernel oil and palm oil); take cod liver oil regularly to supply your body with vitamin A and D; eat fresh fruits and vegetables, preferably organic; eat whole grains and nuts (that have been prepared by soaking, sprouting or sour leavening to begin to neutralize phytic acid and other anti-nutrients); include enzyme-rich lacto-fermented vegetables, fruits, beverages and condiments in your diet on a regular basis; prepare homemade meat stocks from the bones of naturally raised animals; use herb teas; use spring water or filtered water for cooking (and bathing); use unrefined sea salt; use a variety of organic herbs and spices for cooking; use unrefined and natural sweeteners (in only mall amounts); cook in glass, stainless steel, or good quality enamelware.

2. Special Grasses and Medicinal Herbs

Shakyamuni Buddha's second method of special longevity practice was to eat special herbs, plants and botanical substances for their biochemical benefits that would help with health and longevity.

The list of herbs with known special health and longevity benefits is growing on a daily basis, and science is busy researching their properties to determine how to use them. The trick is not just knowing what to consume, but when, how and in what quantities.

Immortal Li already called our attention to the possible life extension properties of Wolfberry (Goji), He Shou Wu (Chinese Knotweed or Fallopia Multiflora) and Reishi (Ganoderma lucidum) mushrooms, which help bolster your immunity. Chinese medicine has identified many other longevity herbs such as Schizandra, Dong Quai (Angelicae Sinensis) and Astragalus, which all have special pharmacological properties for health and healing.

Today we might also add "adaptogens" to the growing list of herbs to be investigated such as American Ginseng (*Panax quinquefolius*), Amalaki (*Emblica officinalis*), Ashwagandha (*Withania somnifera*), Asian Ginseng (*Panax ginseng*), Cordyceps (*Cordyceps sinesis*), Dang Shen (*Codonopsis pilosula*), Eleuthero (*Eleutherococcus senticosus*), Guduchi (*Tinospora cordifolia*), Haritaki (*Terminalia chebula*), Holy Basil (*Ocinum sanctum*), Jiaogulan (*Gynostemna pentaphyllum*), Licorice (*Glycyrrhiza glabra*), Long Pepper (*Piper longum*), Reishi (*Ganoderma ludicum*), Rhodiola (*Rhodiola rosea*), Schisandra (*Schisandra chinensis*), Shatavari (*Asparagus racemosus*), Siberian Ginseng (*Eleutherococcus senticosus*) and Tulsi (*Ocimum sanctum*).

From South America come special herbs such as Pau d'Arco, Cat's Claw, Jergon Sacha, and Suma while North America offers Milk Thistle, Hawthorn berries, and Chaga which "contains the force of actual trees." Even spices, like cinnamon and turmeric (containing Curcumin), have special longevity properties because they can play a role in the important task of managing your blood sugar level, which is implicated in life extension. There are thousands of other helpful herbs that can help your health in various ways, including life extension.

Indian Rasayana practices, geared towards producing longevity, commonly use Ashwaganda and Amalaki, the fruit of a citrus tree and one of the most powerful rejuvenation herbs in Ayurveda. Chyawanprash (whose main ingredient is Amalaki) is also an elaborate Ayurvedic combination of herbs, fruits and minerals you can buy that is especially designed for rejuvenation.

There are a large number of Indian Ayurvedic and Traditional Chinese Medicine anti-aging formulas that have been developed over the ages (but which lack any of the newer adaptogens or other helpful ingredients recently discovered) to help with our human efforts at producing health and longevity. The combination of compounds in these formulas is often quite effective even though the individual compounds often don't have much activity on their own. This is why the avenue of mineral-herbal anti-aging efforts needs to have more research done on how to properly identify and combine useful ingredients to make them more effective and more powerful.

As time marches on the list of helpful longevity herbs or plant substances, such as resveratrol and Curcumin, will grow. The point is that while meditation is essential in seeking longevity (because of its effects on your vital energy) your physical body needs special care and attention as well. For this purpose, special herbal plant substances can help. Special herbal substances can benefit your physical body biochemically so you should certainly use them to stay younger or become younger. You should look into using any anti-aging herbs or plants that have been scientifically discovered to be beneficial for health and longevity. However, while modern science might promote this avenue of assistance it totally ignores the primary emphasis Shakyamuni Buddha and Immortal Li placed on Qi cultivation, so while you should use supplements on the quest for longevity you also need to add meditation to your efforts as well.

3. Special Minerals and Stones

The third practice which Shakyamuni Buddha mentioned was ingesting special metals and minerals to help with life extension, which is a practice that immortality-seeking Taoists also highly recommended. This is not surprising since most people in ancient times were mineral deficient (especially as regards iron and iodine). Mineral deficiency is a great obstacle to life extension since minerals are the necessary building blocks and co-factors in many biochemical reactions. Any deficiencies would therefore be a barrier to life extension efforts.

The easy remedy to mineral deficiencies in the diet is to supplement with some form of easily absorbable minerals. The female Tibetan cultivator Yeshe Tsogyel, who lived well over one hundred years of age, wrote in her autobiography that she imbibed a substance called "chongshi" that she called the "essence of minerals." She mentioned, "I used it in my continued practice of the alchemical metamorphosis of my body-mind," meaning that she relied on a mineral substance for its health benefits.

What was this substance? It was the pitch substance shilajit, which is exuded from the rocks of the Himalayas. It contains at least 85 minerals in ionic form as well as fulvic acid and humic acid, to which are attributed many of its beneficial properties. A related substance available for consumption would be colloidal minerals derived from shale deposits whose toxic metal components, such as aluminum, have been removed.

While minerals are readily absorbed from vegetarian sources such as kelp and green/red superfoods, the products shilajit, colloidal mineral liquids and mineral concentrates (from companies such as Purest Colloids, Trace Minerals Research, Marine Minerals, Goldstake Minerals) provide a more easily assimilable alternative.

Even so, you must remember that minerals by and in themselves do not produce life extension. They only counter deficiencies in your diet and supplement your body's mineral stores so that your biochemical reactions can operate effectively. Supplementation prevents mineral deficiencies and thus in supplying minerals you aid your body's biochemical processes. This is how they affect life extension.

Once again, the real key to life extension is not minerals but meditation. This is why Taoist Lu Dong Bin once said, "As to the five special minerals and eight precious stones, yes they are good but I know that the Path is to cultivate emptiness. If I want to become an immortal, why should I use external herbs? There are much better ways. I can actually produce the wonderful medicinal life essence - Qi - in my own body."

The Taoist Immortal Lu Dong Bin was simply saying that the supreme medicines of longevity are Jing, Qi and Shen (body, life force and spirit). Jing converts into Qi naturally if it isn't lost and then Qi converts into Spirit, or mental force. Your clarity of thought and mind (Shen) certainly depends on the energy state of your body (Qi). Your Spirit (Shen or mental force) depends on your Qi to function. Your body needs to be filled with Qi to stay healthy and live long; if your Qi levels are insufficient you will get sick and experience decline. If you harmonize your Qi, you will save your Spirit. If you can make your Qi and Spirit work together then you can have longevity.

The true path to longevity therefore always involves meditation because of its beneficial effects on both our Qi and Spirit. Minerals just assist the biophysics of the body, made of Jing, to keep it operating harmoniously for this to happen.

4. Mastering Your Breath and Qi

Shakyamuni Buddha said that the fourth type of practice that can lead to longevity is performing breathing exercises, such as pranayama. Pranayama, and in particular the breath retention practices called kumbhaka, can help you to cultivate your Qi and open up your Qi channels. This is why they are commonly identified in eastern traditions as aids to any efforts at life extension.

The *Hatha Yoga Pradipika* of Indian Yoga contains many pranayama techniques, saying "Pranayama should be practiced daily so that impurities are driven out of the body and purification occurs. ... By proper practice of pranayama all your diseases will be eradicated. ... According to some teachers, pranayama alone removes internal impurities and therefore they hold pranayama in esteem and not any other cultivation techniques."

In other words, pranayama will not just help to make your breathing more efficient, but it will help you activate the vital energy life force (Qi) within your body and therefore help to open up the energy channel pathways in all your tissues. Those results will help you live longer.

Various Taoist breathing methods provide similar benefits as well. For instance, the Taoist breathing practices of "spitting out the old (breath) to bring in the new" are basically kumbhaka pranayama methods. All these various breath retention techniques are like using a match to ignite the potential energy in your body (known as kundalini or Yang Qi energy). After you raise this energy and open up your Qi channels some people are said to be able to survive by "eating" air alone.

The most powerful pranayama technique I know of comes from Tibet and is called "9-Bottled Wind Pranayama." Once again it is a kumbhaka or breath retention technique that involves holding your breath nine times.

As you would expect, the purpose is to increase your lung capacity, make your lungs and respiratory processes more efficient (which makes your breathing smoother, deeper and more regular), help open up your Qi channels, and improve the Qi circulation within your body.

The 9-Bottled Wind Pranayama technique involves slowly drawing air into your lungs using an alternate nostril practice technique, fully filling your lungs as much as possible with that air, holding the air deeply inside your lungs for as long as possible while staying relaxed (not tensing any muscles but keeping them as loose as possible), and quickly expelling the air when you can hold it no longer, shooting it out like an arrow.

The 9-Bottled Wind Practice steps are as follows: (1) Sit in an upright position. (2) Visualize your body becoming as clear as crystal. (3) Close your mouth and also close your left nostril completely by pressing your left hand's index finger against the left nostril to shut it. (4) Slowly inhale air deeply into your lungs through your right nostril. The inhalation should consist of a long breath that goes inside you as deep into your abdomen as possible. During your inhalation, visually imagine that your body becomes filled with a bright light that eliminates any internal poisons or obstructions. Continue inhaling as slowly and deeply as possible until you are full and can inhale no longer. (5) Now relax your body as much as possible while holding your trapped breath within. Hold your breath for as long as possible, but use as few muscles as possible to do so. Don't tighten any muscles so that your Qi can start opening up all the tiny energy channels in your body without having to fight muscle tension. (6) When you can hold your breath no longer, exhale it as quickly and forcefully as possible through the other open nostril. Forcefully expel the air out of your body quickly to complete one cycle or round of this exercise. (7) Repeat this exercise of slow inhalation, long retention, and forceful exhalation two more times for a total of three times for the right nostril. All the while the left nostril is kept closed while the active nostril is the right nostril.

(8) Now switch hands so that the right hand's index finger now pinches shut the right nostril while the left remains open. Inhale through your left nostril following the same instructions as before, hold your breath for as long as possible and then forcefully exhale. Repeat this exercise three times for this side of the body. Thus, six repetitions of this exercise will now have

been completed.

(9) When the left and right nostril breathings are both done, extend both your arms out to push on your lap, locking your elbows, and lift up your chest. Inhale slowly through both open nostrils, hold your breath within for as long as possible, and then exhale quickly by shooting the air out from your nostrils when you can't hold the air any longer. Do this for a total of three times.

Altogether nine inhalations and retentions are thereby performed using this simple breath retention technique, which gives rise to the name of 9-step bottled wind practice.

Many people get tired of practicing this technique, so if it is just reduced to inhaling and holding your breath for as long as possible and afterwards exhaling quickly with an expelling force, and doing this as many times as possible during a short pranayama session per day, you will still get most of the benefits. Yogis who practice pranayama to live longer will do many breath retention sessions like this throughout the day, each day trying to beat their best of holding their breath for as long as possible. In this way they gradually open up their Qi channels and lay a strong foundation for longevity.

Another method for "cultivating the breath (Qi)" comes from Japan and is known as the Soma Cream or Duck Egg visualization. It is an inner Qi exercise that Japanese mountain Master Hakuyu taught young Zen master Hakuin when he was passing through the advanced process of Qi channel openings we call the kundalini awakening.

This technique harmonizes all the Qi energy within your body, and Master Hakuyu attributed to this method all his benefits of health and longevity. At age eighty Master Hakuin was still strong and vigorous in both his body and mind, and he also attributed his robust health and vitality to Master Hakuyu's teachings.

The method is very simple and something that you can practice at home on a daily basis if you seek longevity and anti-aging effects.

After asking for instructions, Master Hakuyu told the student Hakuin, "When a student engaged in meditation finds that he is exhausted in body and mind because the four constituent elements of his body are in a state of disharmony, he should gird up his spirit and perform the following visualisation:

"Imagine that a lump of soft butter, pure in colour and fragrance and the size and shape of a duck egg, is suddenly placed on the top of your head. As it begins to slowly melt, it imparts an exquisite sensation, moistening and saturating your head within and without. It continues to ooze down, moistening your shoulders, elbows, and chest; permeating lungs, diaphragm, liver, stomach, and bowels; moving down the spine through the hips, pelvis, and buttocks.

"At that point, all the congestions that have accumulated within the five organs and six viscera, all the aches and pains in the abdomen and other affected parts, will follow the heart as it sinks downward into the lower body. As it does, you will distinctly hear a sound like that of water trickling from a higher to a lower place. It will move lower down through the lower body, suffusing the legs with beneficial warmth, until it reaches the soles of the feet, where it stops.

"The student should then repeat the contemplation. As his vital energy flows downward, it gradually fills the lower region of the body, suffusing it with penetrating warmth, making him feel as if he were sitting up to his navel in a hot bath filled with a decoction of rare and fragrant medicinal herbs that have been gathered and infused by a skilled physician.

"Inasmuch as all things are created by the mind, when you engage in this contemplation, the nose will actually smell the marvellous scent of pure, soft butter; your body will feel the exquisite sensation of its melting touch. Your body and mind will be in perfect peace and harmony. You will feel better and enjoy greater health than you did as a youth of twenty or thirty. At this time, all the undesirable accumulations in your vital organs and viscera will melt away. Stomach and bowels will function perfectly. Before you know it, your skin will glow with health. If you continue to practise the contemplation with diligence, there is no illness that cannot be cured, no virtue that cannot be acquired, no level of sagehood that cannot be reached, no religious practice that cannot be mastered. Whether such results appear swiftly or slowly depends only upon how scrupulously you apply yourself.

"I was a sickly youth, in much worse shape than you are now. I experienced ten times the suffering you have endured. The doctors finally gave up on me. I explored hundreds of cures on my own, but none of them brought me any relief. I turned to the gods for help. Prayed to the deities of both heaven and earth, begging them for their subtle, imperceptible assistance. I was marvellously blessed. They extended me their support and protection. I came upon this wonderful method of soft-butter contemplation. My joy knew no bounds. I immediately set about practising it with total and single-minded determination. Before even a month was out, my troubles had almost totally vanished. Since that time, I've never been the least bit bothered by any complaint, physical or mental."[2]

Master Hakuyu also explained that because of his cultivation, "Even during the months when there are no mountain fruits or nuts for me to gather, and I have no grain to eat, I don't starve. It is all thanks to this contemplation."

There are many other types of breathing practices that can help with the

[2] *Wild Ivy: The Spiritual Autobiography of Zen Master Hakuin*, trans. Norman Waddell (Shambhala Publications, Boston, 1999).

effort to live longer, most of which cultivate your Qi or Qi channels. That's the secret. As seen, the first type are what the yoga schools call kumbhaka (breath retention) pranayama techniques. The second type are Qi balancing techniques, such as taught by Immortal Li and mountain master Hakuyu. You can find more on these techniques in my book *Nyasa Yoga*.

5. Cultivate Your Fluids and Saliva

The fifth method of practice was to cultivate one's water element (fluids) and saliva, which actually refers to cultivating your hormones by generating and swallowing a special sweet salivary hormone that is released during advanced stages of meditation when your Qi channels begin to open in your head and brain. Sometimes a little is released during sexual intercourse when the Qi channels in the head start to open because of the vital energies entering into the cranium because of this activity.

The esoteric science behind this is as follows. At a certain advanced stage of meditation practice the salivary glands start secreting a sweet liquid that is often compared to wine. You cannot force it to be secreted because it only appears for a short while due to excellent meditation work.

This sweet salivary hormone greatly assists with health and longevity. Many cultivation schools say it helps expel toxins from the body, softens and strengthens bones and tendons, and helps to rejuvenate your body in general. Therefore, they say, its ingestion (swallowing) leads to longevity.

The *Hatha Yoga Pradipika* poetically refers to it saying, "The Yogi who drinks the pure stream of nectar from the head will become free of disease, attain longevity, and their body will soften and become as beautiful as a lotus stem." You can also find mention of it in Nan Huai-chin's *Tao and Longevity* and Swami Satyananda Saraswati's *A Systematic Course in the Ancient Tantric Techniques of Yoga and Kriya*. It is also recognized in the western alchemy text, the *Atalanta Fugiens* of Michael Maier. Its appearance is the legendary "Fountain of Youth" said to restore the youth of anyone who drinks its waters, or the Pool of Bethesda in the New Testament whose waters produce healing when stirred. Basically this sweet tasting "dew" is the ambrosia, soma, grail wine, or legendary fountain of youth that is said to lead to immortality (long life). Only meditation and other spiritual practices can produce it.

Unfortunately, ordinary people who do not practice meditation enough cannot experience it, and therefore cannot practice this technique unless the sweet saliva hormone appears. However, by using visualization practices that focus on the glands of the body, which will bring Qi to those regions due to mental concentration held at those points, the endocrine system of the body can become activated to help you reach longevity. This method is to visualize your glands as they are located in your body and to spin your Qi within them and around hem.

Immortal Li also taught that people who wanted to live longer should make use of a regular regimen of stimulating and then swallowing their saliva combined with breathing practices. Why is this helpful?

Swallowing your saliva will help your Qi descend to your lower belly, but before swallowing saliva you must first collect it. The method for collecting and then swallowing saliva is to do the following, which also exercises the muscles in your mouth:

Place your tongue against the inside of your left cheek and then move it, in a rolling motion, to the right cheek by passing over the front of the upper teeth (and gums) and then continue downwards in front of the lower teeth (and gums) until you reach the left cheek again. Do this eighteen times and then repeat the same procedure eighteen times in the other direction starting with the right cheek and moving to the left. This practice of moving the tongue thirty-six times will accumulate saliva in the mouth, and then one should swallow it while visualizing that your Qi descends into your lower abdomen.

In addition to exercising the tongue and preparing the practitioner for the higher yogic practice of ingesting Qi in the air and swallowing it, this practice has many other benefits.

Stimulating, collecting and swallowing your saliva, as a means of cultivation, is commonly taught in Taoism especially in conjunction with the pranayama practices of drawing in good Qi and expelling bad Qi - "spitting out the old (breath) to bring in the new." These pranayama practices are basically the idea of breath retention where you draw in air, hold it until you can no longer, and then expel it quickly and forcefully.

6. Absorb the Essences of the Sun and Moon

The sixth method of longevity practice Shakyamuni Buddha mentioned was to absorb the energies of the sun and moon, which means the pure Yin and Yang energies from celestial bodies and the environment, in order to supplement your own Yin and Yang Qi energies. You basically try to absorb into your body the energy from the sun, moon, earth, stars, or planets.

To do this you can envision the light energies from the sun or planets embracing your entire person, reaching inside you as far as the bottom of the abdomen in the pelvis (visually imagine the energies filling your whole body), giving yourself the feeling of being completely illuminated within and without. After you imagine that your body becomes filled with energy, you must imagine that your whole body become luminous and shines brightly with these energies.

You particularly want the energies to reach your abdomen and fill your lower belly called the dantian or Elixir Field in Chinese medicine, qigong and martial arts. Immortal Li said that you might rub your belly on a daily basis to help bathe it in Qi vital energy (concentrating on that area mentally while doing so in order to bring Qi to the region), but the important point is to draw your energy down into this area and keeping that region warm so that the Qi can open up all the energy channels in the intestinal tissues through a slow permeation process we might call Qi soaking.

Other practices for absorbing energy from the sun and moon and stars or other planets do not involve imaginary visualizations. With these methods you must physically gaze at the sun, moon or stars (such as the Big Dipper or Polestar) in order to try to absorb their essences. To succeed with this method requires special conditions of time and place, but some individuals do succeed at it despite the difficulties. They can then begin to live without food and survive on just these energies alone.

The first method of actual absorption, from Chinese Taoism, is that you inhale as you "breathe" into your body the sun's energy through the crown point of your skull (the very top of your head). You pull the energy of the sun into the center of your brain, and then into your entire head area including the maxillary glands that produce saliva. Gather the energy into your mouth and mix it with the saliva accumulating there. Visualize the energy condensing into a golden ball and then swallow this ball of Yang Qi down into your lower belly as you exhale. Repeat this process three or four times and then focus your breathing on your lower abdomen to feel the warmth of the sun residing there.

As an alternative, you can also stand in the sunshine and feel the sun pouring into you from the top of your head and filling up the entire body, accumulating inside you just as sand flows into the base of an hour-glass to fill it. When you feel that your whole body is filled with this solar energy then stay in that state lightly holding onto the energy, feeling it everywhere, while letting go of your thoughts.

The second type of solar absorption, from ancient India, is known as sun eating. In this case it is a strict practice of gradually absorbing sunlight into your eyes at the safest (lowest UV-index) times of the day, which are at sunrise and sunset when the sun is low on the horizon. The method can only be practiced within the first hour after sunrise and right before sunset because otherwise you will risk damaging your eyes. You should never stare at or focus on the sun when doing it or you will hurt your eyes.

You must also be *standing barefoot* while performing this practice, standing on the actual earth. Why? Since this method involves absorbing solar Yang Qi energies you must be grounded to the Yin Qi of the earth to complete an energetic circuit.

To practice this sun eating technique you should begin with only 10 seconds the first day and increase by 10 seconds each day. Never practice it for more than a few minutes. Once you start doing this you will start feeling full of energy, which will help to supplement your Qi and open up your Qi channels. Some people who do this earn the ability to be able to live off the energy alone and therefore can radically decrease the amount of food they need to survive. Some can actually survive on just this energy alone.

If you use any technique of trying to absorb Yang Qi you should also match it with the practice of absorbing the Yin Qi energy of the moon. The best results for absorbing Yin energy are achieved around the full moon period of each month when the lunar light is brightest. At that time you can feel you are absorbing/pulling the Yin Qi energy into your body through the top of your head as we did with the first solar Qi method, and then also absorb lunar moonlight though the eyes, pulling it into the brain and sending it to the back of your head. An alternative is to pull the lunar area into your heart-chest area.

There are also techniques for absorbing the energy of the planet Venus when it is visible and other planets as well (especially when they are stationary), but they are all based on the same basic techniques. The idea is to augment your own Qi from the Qi of a greater celestial source, and to use that extra energy to help transform your body by opening up the energy channels in all the atomic bonds within it. This will create an extremely healthy body.

7. Mantra and Special Cultivation Techniques

The seventh special method of longevity practice was the spiritual exercise of reciting mantras.

In most every religion, and especially in eastern spiritual traditions, there are special mantras (and prayers) that request help from higher beings for various matters, including requests for help at curing sickness or life extension. For instance, the mantra for Immortal Li's tradition that requests Heaven's aid for health, longevity and spiritual progress is "Ohm Ah Hung Ah Hung."

The way Heaven helps after higher beings hear mantras, if Heaven helps at all, is through the intercession of spiritual beings supplying thoughts to help you solve problems or extra energy to help open up your Qi channels. This happens to virtuous people engaging in spiritual practice when they have enough merit (such as from doing good deeds or making a great vow to change your behavior, such as becoming vegetarian). The idea of asking for the blessing of someone else's energy is basically a supplementation remedy.

There are also mantra practices that will help you to quiet your mind, which ultimately leads to the arising of your deep Qi energies and thus once again the opening of your Qi channels that is necessary for super longevity.

For life extension purposes the most effective mantra practices are "Nyasa" practices that help transform and preserve your body. Most people have never heard of Nyasa practices but they combine mantra recitations with visualization efforts on sections of the body while you try to feel and visualize the energy (Qi) within those areas in order to open up the surrounding energy channels that form the substrate of the physical body.

An individual practicing Nyasa selects a part of their body, focuses on it with concentration while visualizing that it is either shining with light or changes color, recites a mantra as if from within that location (thus vibrating it) in order to move his Qi to that area and open up the Qi channels in that immediate region, and tries to physically *feel* that area being focused upon or the sensations within it. He then continues doing so until one by one he has done this for all the parts and sections of the body.

There are many types of Nyasa practice with some being very complex and elaborate. Many Vajrayana practices in Tibet are actually Nyasa practice in disguise, including some deity yoga methods.

Two famous "dharma" techniques related to the Nyasa practices are the white skeleton visualization practice of Shakyamuni Buddha and the fire skeleton visualization method of Mahavira, the founder of Jainism.

The white skeleton visualization practice can be done if you are either sitting on a chair, on meditation cushions or lying flat on your back. There are over thirty different variations of the practice that all energize and raise your Qi levels so that your Qi channels start opening.

To practice, in whatever position you have chosen, first take a couple of deep breaths and release any tension you feel in your body.

Starting from your left big toe, begin to visualize that you no longer have flesh on the foot and that your left big toe bones shine with a dazzling white light. First visualize the bones of your left big toe, then all of the toes on your left foot. Then switch sides to visualize the bones of the right big toe shining with a dazzling white light and then all of the toes of your right foot shining brightly.

Next, do the same for all the remaining bones of your left foot, and then your right foot. Next the bones of your left ankle and then right ankle (while keeping the other bones shining that you already did). Going higher proceed to both left lower-leg bones and then right lower-leg bones (the tibia and fibula in both legs).

Continue like this visualizing all the meat being stripped off your bones and all the exposed bones shining with a bright white light. Try to feel the energy in that body region as you do this because the practice will bring energy to each body section in turn.

Gradually work your way up your body, visualizing that your body is just a set of bones without flesh, the bones are shining brightly, and you can feel the energy in those regions. Eventually you will reach the head and can end with a visualization of your skull shining with a bright white light.

Once the visualization of your entire skeleton is complete, try to maintain it until you feel that your Qi has become distributed in an evenly balanced manner everywhere. Whenever you feel any sensations that arise just note them but don't grasp onto them or cling to them. In fact, if you feel any energy then try to stir it up to make it bigger because stimulated energy that becomes active will open up more channels in the region. Also, try to maintain a joyful state of mind as you perform this entire visualization because joy gives rise to positive energies, and thus raises Yang Qi instead of Yin Qi.

After you visualize your entire body as a set of brightly shining white bones, visualize that they all become dust that is instantly blown away and the only thing remaining is empty space that you cannot hold onto. In other words, imagine that now you are nothing but empty space. Ignore the energy feelings that arise while in this state because if you interfere with those energy flows you will thwart the efforts of your Qi to open up Qi channels.

As for a similar technique used by the Jains, you imagine that there is a large fiery lotus flower inside you at the level of your navel, bright red in color, that is burning with red flames that extend upwards and protrude out the top of the center of your head. At the level of your heart, you then imagine an inverted lotus flower made of fire that is also bright red in color. The flame that flows between these two lotus flowers is imagined to energize your entire body turning it entirely into red glowing ashes.

After you can visualize your entire body as red and filled with this fiery energy, imagine that a strong wind blows off all the ashes and then a heavy rain falls from above and washes all the ashes away so that a pure soul or transparent body remains seated at your spot. Then let go of all visions and rest your mind by imaging that you are empty space that holds onto nothing.

Yet another visualization technique from tantric yoga is to imagine that your body becomes entirely energized by red fire energy, just as seen in pictures of the Tibetan deity Vajrayogini, and once accomplished you again release the visualization practice and let your mind rest in emptiness without attaching to any of the Qi sensations that arise within.

All these techniques work to open up the Qi channels of your body. Using visualization as the energizing, vitalizing or innervation mechanism since it moves your Qi, you progressively increase the size of your body region affected until you feel your Qi moving all over. You always try to stimulate, energize or stir it up using this method. Once you reach a state of harmonious fullness, you let go of attaching (clinging) to those sensations and mentally rest in emptiness so that your Qi channels will open naturally (due to the Qi that has just been activized into moving and opening your channels).

The cultivation of your Qi and channels is what leads to super life extension.

8. Meditation

The eighth method of longevity practice, according to Shakyamuni Buddha, was simply the practice of meditation.

You have to meditate nearly every day in order to obtain the benefits of opening up your Qi channels to extend your life span. Many methods of meditation are possible which you can learn about in my books, *The Little Book of Meditation* and *Meditation Case Studies*. Vipassana practice, as taught by many western meditation teachers, is also a good start.

It is said that Immortal Li, when he had time, would sit up straight with eyes closed and his hands in his lap, at times not moving for hours. This of course was the practice of meditation.

9. Sexual Intercourse with Discipline

The ninth method of practice is often misunderstood as Shakyamuni mentioned that individuals could use sexual intercourse (sexual technique) to help with life extension. The explanation is as follows.

Almost everyone who has had sex has at one time or another has felt energy move inside him/her that could not be attributed to nerve stimulation or emotions. This is actually the activization of Qi, or life force, within the body that can be stimulated or activated through sex. The entire idea of sexual intercourse as a longevity practice is that a man and woman should engage in sex without the man ejaculating to experience semen loss (female orgasm is allowed) so as to move their Qi and thereby open up the Qi channels. For sexual cultivation, one learns to master the physical and energetic stimuli and responses of intercourse.

Different positions and tempos during love-making can cause your Qi to arise and initiate particular Qi movements that open up different Qi channels. When enough of the right Qi channels open this will extend your longevity. This route of using sex to open up Qi channels is used in some spiritual schools (Chinese Taoism, Vajrayana Buddhism and the Maithuna practices of Hindu kaula tantra yoga) to help transform the physical body. However, the effectiveness of the efforts decline tremendously if a man ejaculates because he will lose both his Jing and Qi in the process. Those are the essences one must build up and retain in order to open up one's Qi channels and achieve longevity.

The ancient Chinese medical text, *The Yellow Emperor's Classic of Internal Medicine*, recounts:

"I [the Yellow Emperor] have heard that men in ancient times lived to be over 200 years old, the men of middle antiquity commonly lived to be 120 years old, but the men of our time rarely live to reach even 30 years of age. Too many men nowadays are also suffering illness and disease. Why do you think this is so?" His enlightened female teacher answered him, "It is because they ejaculate too frequently and emit their Jing (semen) indiscriminately when they make love. It is cutting off the root foundation of their lives. How can they then expect to live long?"

She also told the Emperor, "When a couple practices lovemaking correctly the man will remain healthy and youthful rather than become depleted, and because of the benefitting Qi flow the woman will avoid a hundred diseases. Done properly, both the man and woman will enjoy sex thoroughly and at the same time increase their physical strength rather than deplete it through exhaustion. However, if they don't know how to practice lovemaking correctly then sexual intercourse can be harmful to their health. The key is not to lose your Qi during the process. As a good guideline, one should stop when the female is completely satisfied and the male is not yet exhausted."

Within the Jing of the body resides its generative force, for it can create a new life, and within the Qi of the body resides the life force of the organism. You don't want to lose these through sex. Our vitality is basically adequate in the human body but can dissipate because of too much sexual indulgence or emotional excesses. If Jing and Qi become exhausted due to sexual loss then one should remedy the loss through restraint until their levels are gradually restored. Due to the restraint of refraining from sex, little by little those essences will accumulate and one's energy will return.

In *Think and Grow Rich*, the famous writer Napoleon Hill wrote,

"I discovered, from the analysis of over 25,000 people, that men who succeed in an outstanding way, seldom do so before the age of forty, and more often they do not strike their real pace until they are well beyond the age of fifty. This fact was so astounding that it prompted me to go into the study of its cause most carefully.

"This study disclosed the fact that the major reason why the majority of men who succeed do not begin to do so before the age of forty to fifty, is their tendency to dissipate their energies through over-indulgence in physical expression of the emotion of sex. The majority of men never learn that the urge of sex has other possibilities, which far transcend in importance that of mere physical expression. The majority of those who make this discovery, do so after having wasted many years at a period when the sex energy is at its height, prior to the age of forty-five to fifty. This usually is followed by noteworthy achievement."[3]

---

[3] *Think and Grow Rich*, Napoleon Hill, (Ballantine Books, New York, 1960).

Napoleon Hill's observation speaks to the fact that after men stop squandering their Jing and Qi they finally start making great accomplishments in life, and this also applies to the practice of meditation for spiritual progress and life extension.

10. Matching with Earthly & Heavenly Conditions

The last method of practice that Shakyamuni Buddha mentioned was to match oneself with heavenly and earthly transformations in order to live longer. In terms of earthly conditions this refers to the influences of the four seasons as well as any local geographical Feng Shui energies (the Chinese science of geomancy) and conditions. In terms of heavenly conditions this refers to various astronomical phenomena (which also means astrological phenomena) since their energies affect the Qi flowing within your subtle body.

All of these influences affect the Yin and Yang energies of the environment in which you live, and as the recipient of those energies (since you live within them) they can help you or hurt you depending upon whether they are harmful or helpful and whether you accord with them or against them. The idea of cultivation is to go along with nature rather than fight against or oppose the momentum of greater forces. As in the martial arts, one should use these external energies to help you accomplish your objectives.

The idea of matching yourself with earthly and cosmic conditions is therefore to use these energies to help in the process of Qi channel openings since this ultimately leads to longevity, and thus you want to be swimming with the tide of these energies in a helpful fashion rather than fighting against them.

Astronomical influences, especially the energies of the sun and of the moon as it proceeds through its phases, have a strong effect on your subtle body (Qi). Just as the moon governs the rhythms, cycles and activity of the tides it affects your thoughts and emotions through its influences on the Qi of your body and any liquid elements inside it such as your hormones.

The phases of the moon typically have a strong effect on your energy levels, which is why religious holidays across the world are often timed according to the phases of the moon. This is done to capture the benefit of some of those energies.

The earthly march of the four seasons also affects your body in a regular cycle that you must learn to match up with. The four seasons necessitate different living rules for the different parts of the year, such as Immortal Li Qingyun's advice that you should never skip breakfast in winter and never eat too late in summer. There are many rules or principles for warding off disease that have to do with recognizing the influences or energies of the seasons and then acting accordingly. Normally, we just call this "wise living."

This method of achieving life extension also refers back to the original Taoist ideas that the orbits of the planets in heaven last forever, and a human being could achieve a similar longevity if he matched himself with these immortal (perennially regular) earthly and cosmic transformations. This means matching yourself with the influence of the earthly seasons and the cosmic energies reaching us from the stars that produce worldly influences and effect our fortunes.

Chinese culture identifies these forces using "ten heavenly stems" and "twelve earthly branches" while other cultures use planets or refer to the "five elements" (earth, wind, fire, water, space) to categorize them. However they designate them, most cultures suggest that you don't fight against these forces but adapt yourself to them and the conditions they create to live longer. In our case we just want to use these powerful energies whenever possible to supplement our Qi and open up our Qi channels. This is why spiritual cultivators in China often live in special holy mountains. The strong Qi of those areas can be used to supplement cultivators' own energies and help penetrate and open up the energy channels within their bodies.

An ancient Chinese saying runs, "The sage takes his signs from the movements of Heaven and Earth; who knows the principles? He accords with the principles of Yin and Yang by following their seasonal activity. He follows the fullness and emptiness of Heaven and Earth, taking them as his constant." Those interested in longevity should do likewise. They should observe the weather and the seasons to adjust their clothing, diet and other activities accordingly. If they are proficient in understanding the influences of astronomical phenomena, they can use them as well.

Even the Indian medical school of Ayurveda, the "science of longevity," says that you should live in harmony with the external environment. "Accord with nature and longevity comes" does not just refer to the principles of aging and biochemistry, but to the matching with heavenly and earthly energies.

SIDDHA MEDICINE

In addition to ten methods for life extension taught by Shakyamuni Buddha and the Indian medical system of Ayurveda (which offers rasayana remedies using foods, herbs and minerals), the Siddha medical system from Tamil India also suggest anti-aging and rejuvenation (*kaya-karpam*) methods.

The Siddha road speaks of taking herbs, ingesting calcinated powders made from metals and minerals, and taking muppu (a "universal salt" similar to shilajit) for physical rejuvenation and longevity. Naturally these are roads of assistance that Shakyamuni already covered.

Like Shakyamuni and the Chinese Taoists, the Siddha medicine road to prolonging life also speaks about the need for sexual restraint to avoid the loss of Jing (semen), thus conserving male secretions, while the meaning of such restraint in every tradition is not to indiscriminately lose Jing *and* Qi through emission. And as with Buddhism and Taoism, the Siddha road to prolonging life also involves controlled breathing and yoga practices.

Once again, all these practices work at opening up your Qi channels.

SYNOPSIS

Shakyamuni Buddha recommended ten practices to promote health and extend the human life span, including supplementation of nutrients from plants and minerals; supplementation of energy from extraterrestrial bodies and cosmic processes; supplementation of assistance from higher powers through mantras; stimulation of internal energy through physical and mental exercises as well as controlled sexual intercourse.

The important point to recognize from these methods is that they typically duplicate the recommendations of Taoism *and* modern nutritional science. For instance, when you eat special foods, herbs or minerals the longevity approach you are taking is a supplementation method that assists your body's biochemical processes. You are basically supplying the body with the right nutrients for growth and repair so that you can live longer. This addresses the Jing or physical structure of the body, and through that its Qi or life force energy.

Throughout the Buddhist methods, supplementation is critical just as we found with Taoism. Here we find supplementation of both Jing and Qi. You might supplement your Qi energy using the borrowed energies of the sun and moon, or make use of the special Qi energies of the earth and various cosmic processes. Mantra practice or prayer requests help from higher powers, which is a request for Qi supplementation energies as well.

When your Qi becomes full due to supplementation, it will start to open up your Qi channels, which is essentially a process of detoxification (easily noticed because it is accompanied by warmth) that will push harmful poisons out of your body. This is why regular herbal methods of detoxification to help cleanse and purify your body can *greatly* help with the goals of health, longevity and even spiritual practice.

Many methods can be used to electrify, excite, invigorate, stimulate, animate, trigger or vitalize your Qi (however you wish to describe it) so that it starts opening up your Qi channels. Pranayama breathing practices, visualization practices and sexual intercourse accomplish this as does the right types of stretching exercise that also move your energy. Lastly, there is the admonition not to lose your Qi in the first place, but to preserve it so that during meditation practice there is sufficient quantity enough that its accumulated mass can begin to open up your channels.

Television and SciFi movies paint a fantasy picture that super longevity will come about in the future from medical pills or special equipment. Almost no one talks about the road of cultivating our life force essence itself, Qi.

However, that is what you have to do for real longevity. Exercising to stretch your Qi channels open will help longevity efforts and so will biochemical assistance for your body that comes from ingesting special plants, minerals and herbs. Meditation practice that ends up augmenting your Qi can also produce a big impact too. Meditation practice can definitely help you look younger and live longer.

If you want to live a very long life you must open up your Qi channels, cultivate the Qi of your body and create an inner independent life whose own longevity, due to more purified energetic elements, can be used to support the physical body to keep it alive. If you achieve that inner spiritual body of Qi you become an Immortal as the Taoists and Shakyamuni have taught. Immortal Li actually achieved this state in order to be able to live so long, but few people know this since they are unfamiliar with the genuine results of spiritual cultivation.

If you don't achieve this inner Qi body cultivation then no amount of pharmaceuticals, foods, drugs or exercises will help you live incredibly longer. You can achieve life extension through these other methods, but not incredible life extension without Qi cultivation. This is why all your life extension efforts should always be accompanied by meditation and other spiritual practices that affect the Qi of your body.

At the very end of the day the quest for health and longevity will require wisdom (understanding these principles), discipline (to follow methods that offer the best chances of success), merit (blessing) and meditation practice.

Chapter 5
Lessons From The "Blue Zones"

In 2004 author Dan Buettner teamed up with National Geographic to investigate places in the world where the residents boasted a high level of centenarians, people who lived to be over one hundred years old. He called these areas "Blue Zones," which included locations such as Okinawa (Japan), Sardinia (Italy), Loma Linda, California (which contained a long-lived group of Seventh-day Adventists), Icaria (Greece) and Nicoya Peninsula (Costa Rica).

In these Blue Zones centenarians are found at a proportion many times greater than elsewhere. The residents have generally long life expectancies and low rates of middle age mortality. They typically live long lives, but enjoy happy lives of quality.

The results of Buettner's investigations into the hows and whys behind these pockets of super longevity were published in his *New York Times* best-seller, *The Blue Zones*. In it he reports upon the principles he derived for how people can live longer, healthier lives. The answers that he found are surprisingly similar to the Taoist and Buddhist teachings, and they accord with recommendations logically derived from addressing the modern theories of aging.

Why is it that people in some parts of the world live much longer than others? If we study the habits of people from places where residents commonly live to be over one hundred then we will surely find some secrets of longevity. Buettner's findings were totally independent of knowing the teachings of the Taoists and Buddhists, but you will surprisingly find the exact same longevity principles cherished by these traditions as well as an overlap of shared longevity techniques. The Blue Zones study is our opportunity to not just view the habits of long life span societies using the lens of modern science, but we can also use it to examine the conclusions about longevity from the standpoint of eastern views on spirituality and cultivating your life.

In studying the cultures of the Blue Zone locations Buettner discovered six common characteristics that he believed contributed to their relatively high rate of centenarians and relatively low level of disease.

First, people tended to put family ahead of other concerns, such as money or career (just as you might find in typical eastern cultures).

Second, the centenarians were socially active and integrated into their communities. They were respected members of society as you also typically find in the east where elders are revered.

Third, most of the communities could be classified as semi-vegetarian because most longevity diets were not based on meat but on plant sources.

Fourth, junk food was marginalized just as nutritional science constantly recommends.

Fifth, beans (legumes), rather than wheat or other grains, were the food most commonly consumed by the longest-lived residents in these communities.

Lastly, the residents in these communities were found to be always moving. Constant physical activity, even as simple as walking up and down stairs in order to fetch an item, was an inseparable part of life. (Referencing Immortal Li's life, Blue Zone seniors were found to be exercising by just moving around, so they were actually maintaining their Qi flow and flexibility by exercising without knowing it.)

These six longevity principles were the ones most frequently found across separate longevity communities. They harken back to Immortal Li Qingyun's eastern Taoist teachings and have commonalities with Buddhist teachings as well.

THE BLUE ZONES

In his book, *The Blue Zones*, Buettner summarized nine large principles which he believed were the most important ones responsible for notable life extension. Taken together, these nine principles impact the topic of longevity holistically rather than from just a single angle such as the role played by nutrition.

Here are the nine drivers of longevity he discovered, which are the nine habits to consider adopting if you definitely want to live longer:

1. Maintaining Spiritual Practice

First, those who lived longest were regularly involved with spiritual practices such as religious services, so Buettner concluded that there is a definite, positive benefit to the regular practice of devotion, reverence and staying ritualistic with your beliefs. Science has found through other studies confirming evidence that attending faith-based services adds years to one's life expectancy.

Perhaps the regularity of worship across the holidays and seasons is what helps you keep going, but the ancient Taoists had a different take on the matter. Ages ago the Chinese Taoists also discovered there were great benefits to worship, prayer and religion both on a community and personal level. This is because spiritual practice has the basic ability to help people unify their spirit and cultivate their Qi through the avenue of devotional sincerity. In other words, devotion (such as seen in Hindu bhakti or Christian devotional prayer) produces definite changes in your Qi and Shen, your soul and spirit, your Qi and mind. Because these components of your personality are affected in a beneficial fashion by reverential devotion your Qi channels open, your Qi flows better and this results in greater longevity.

This Taoist conclusion on the importance of ritualistic devotion was the result of profound learning and observation. While the idea of regular spiritual practice results in religious rites, the beneficial basis is actually related to the transformational function of the spiritual life on your soul energy, life force or Qi.

2. Lowering Stress Levels

Second, the world's longest-lived people follow gentle routines to help them shed stress, which is another reason to learn meditation. The gentle routines Buettner found among centenarians might be as simple as adopting a slower pace of life that avoids excessive worries, or taking restful vacations and getting enough quality sleep on a regular basis.

This is, of course, something that Immortal Li would readily recommend.

Downtime helps to reduce internal inflammation, which is a precursor of disease, and gives your body a chance to rest and return to experiencing what is supposed to be its normal Qi circulation. Most people look rested and refreshed after the holidays or a relaxing vacation, and that periodic downtime of renewal is good for longevity.

Everyone has different routines they use to deal with excessive stresses and pressures. Napoleon, for instance, would mentally put all his worries in a drawer before he went to sleep at night resolving to only open up the worry drawer in the morning. That is how he mentally dealt with the stresses of managing an empire.

There is no doubt that stress management – even something as simple as listening to classical music, watching a comedy or unwinding through yoga in order to relax – reduces high blood pressure and gives people more control over their lives and emotions. These activities are beneficial to your health and longevity.

Some people handle adverse negative events by preventing overreaction. They develop strategies such as learning to say, "So what?" since bad things can be good and good things can be bad. Immortal Li loved to recite a daily chant containing the words, "Only today is today" because it reminded him that you will still be in good shape after so many sufferings and trials. He warned us not to be too sad, worried or depressed since in this way we lose Qi from our bodies.

If you want to live longer then learn how to live according to the seasons. Learn how to take a break, eliminate stress, relax and enjoy yourself. Go slower, be more optimistic and learn meditation since it is a form of mental resting. Meditating regularly will help you learn relaxation and deal with the unavoidable stresses of life. Because it raises your vital energy, it will help you look younger and feel younger too.

Studies also show that meditation improves your coping abilities. It raises your threshold for feeling the onset of stress after which negative emotions arise. As Immortal Li said, don't fall into greed, anger, bitter sadness or become vexed by hatred and other excessive emotions or desires. Don't get caught up in the worrying chaos of the world and try to diminish your harmful desires and anxieties if you want to live longer.

3. Having a Life Purpose

Third, the Blue Zones study found that those who lived longest usually had a definite life purpose they tended to, such as volunteering for good causes or caring for children and grandchildren. Another way of saying it is that the longest-lived individuals were engaged in purposeful living.

We have all heard the stories of individuals who worked hard all their lives, retired and then died quickly. Their great folly was consuming the greater portion of their lives making a living for money rather than fulfilling a personal mission of living purposefully, which keeps most people going. Full of sound and fury, most lives lived signify nothing. There is little accomplishment in terms of the service of helping others or impacting the greater community, state, country or world in a beneficial manner. People rarely leave a legacy of good deeds. However, for those who have a life purpose and are engaged in purposeful living they are usually greeted by more well-being and longevity to reward their efforts.

Until they have a life purpose most people feel they are not complete. Remember, living itself is not a life purpose. What you consciously do with life, with your efforts, is living out your life purpose.

What can you offer the world? What goals are worthy of your money, time, energy and efforts? What activities are worthy of you expending your

Qi, your very life essence? What do you want to be remembered for after death? What is it that you want people to be reading on your tomb stone? How would you like your obituary to read? What positive impact do you want to make? These are questions that will help you determine a life purpose.

It turns out that engaging in a purposeful life of ongoing activity (other than just your career) adds years of well-being to a normal life span. Unfortunately most people are working jobs they dislike to pay their bills, and in that case they should live out their life purpose through extracurricular activities outside of work. Whether it is a family role, community role, recreational role, or charitable and philanthropic role, having a sense of life purpose extends longevity.

Don't be walking about in the world as if alive but not living. Don't cut yourself off from inner joy, happiness and purpose and deny yourself by doing something different than what you know you should be doing. If you want to live longer then try to find that inner life purpose. The happiness and contentment you find will help to cultivate your Qi and help you live longer even if there are no monetary rewards to your decision.

Surrendering to a purpose greater than oneself is actually a similar idea to devotion or religious practice. It will cultivate your Qi and spirit and you may help win the benefits of longevity in return.

4. Maintaining Family Life

Fourth, Buettner found that those who lived longest stayed positively engaged with their family life, which was important for many reasons. The unity of a group committed to the welfare of its members helps to extend everyone's life spans, so in this light there are great benefits to staying committed to a life partner, investing in your children and grandchildren, and working to ensure the continuity of the generations as a group. On the other hand, when family members take a passive attitude to their relationships and offer minimal support to the family, the idea of a family is just a shelter or roof under which people all live together. This doesn't have any benefit to the path of longevity.

As economies deteriorate, it will be more common for multiple generations to continue living under one roof, which will require that we learn better family management skills. You will be able to help at these tasks only if you remain healthy. Furthermore, as you get older various restrictions may arise that will affect your roles in family life, but there are still ways to help family members in need, support the family as a cohesive unit, help maintain its stability and harmony, and help it move toward success through discipline.

For longer living, Buettner found that we should basically stay close to our family if we are older and if younger we should keep the elderly close. Maintaining these bonds helps to extend the life.

5. Maintaining Social Engagement

Fifth, the longest-lived people in these longevity communities also chose to associate with others in social circles that supported healthy behaviors and where people helped one another. They didn't sever their relationships with their community or withdraw from society. Staying engaged with and committed to a larger social network are reasons they lived longer. In other words, their community helped them keep going.

For instance, in the book *Outliers*, Malcolm Gladwell wrote about a group of Italians called the Rosetans that had moved to Pennsylvania and who were healthier and lived longer lives than average. What he found was that the Rosetans had created a powerful protective social structure that shielded them from worldly pressures, and it was due to this beneficial social shield that they were healthier and living longer than others.

Typically, as we age the roles we play in life will change. People need to substitute new roles for the ones that they lose over time but still stay socially active in the family and community. Most of the centenarians that Buettner studied avoided the fate of loneliness by maintaining a life of positive social interactions. This definitely increases one's longevity.

Many people don't know that one of the reasons Christianity became successful rather than die out in its infancy was exactly because early Christian followers took care of one another in a community setting of beneficial, helpful relationships. The community of support being offered was one of the biggest attractions to Christianity. Therefore if you want to live longer, as you age continue volunteering and staying active with community service to help yourself keep going.

6. Engaging in Regular Physical Exercise

Sixth, Buettner found that the longest-lived people always seemed to be engaged in regular moderate physical activity. They were not taking exercise classes or lifting weights, but were basically doing very simple things that kept them moving all the time. Their environments were always requiring them to unconsciously move about and undertake physical activity, nudging them to move without their having to think about it.

Studies actually show you only need a moderate amount of exercise to stay healthy, and the centenarians Buettner studied were not working out at the gym, running on treadmills or running marathons. As stated, they were just living life with constant movement.

Simple movement activities such as walking or tending to a garden are just fine to provide this movement as are gentle exercises like Tai chi, stretching and yoga. All these gentle exercises help you to retain your flexibility (a maintenance strategy), move your Qi, and thus keep the Qi life force within your body flowing.

Movement will definitely add to anyone's life expectancy, so if you want to live longer then just move.

7. Moderate Drinking and Special Foods

Seventh, the Blue Zones study showed that most long-lived community residents regularly consumed some special local food or drink – such as red wine, sauerkraut or yoghurt (which contain probiotics) – that had notable benefits for life extension. As noted elsewhere, the types of food that might help with longevity would certainly vary by location.

One particular Buettner finding was that moderate drinkers (especially red wine drinkers) outlived non-drinkers. Perhaps this is due to the resveratrol content within wine, alcohol's beneficial effects on blood circulation, or the fact that alcohol lowers stress levels (and the hormone cortisol) that puts aging wear and tear on the body.

In any case, as Immortal Li advised your drinking should remain moderate. Just as Shakyamuni Buddha pointed out, it can be one of the many foods, herbs and minerals you add to your diet that can assist with life extension efforts. It is best to derive these benefits through simple foods rather than supplements but supplements can play a great role in your efforts at anti-aging too.

8. Maintaining Moderate Calorie Intake

Eighth, scientific studies consistently show that calorie restriction, meaning just a moderate intake of food calories rather than always fully packing your stomach during meals, can extend life spans. Naturally this harkens back to the benefits found with intermittent fasting.

The Blue Zones researchers found that centenarians usually stop eating when their stomach is 80% full, which the Taoists already explained conserved your Qi energy since not all of it was then being diverted to digestion. The Yoga schools stress this fact as well.

If you want to live longer then don't overeat. Don't always stuff yourself until you are full, and don't fill yourself with useless calories or junk food that is sugar-laden. A disciplined diet and eating the right amount of food is greatly responsible for increased longevity.

9. Keeping to Plant-Based Diets

Ninth, it was found that the longest-lived people consumed what w primarily a plant-based diet. Organic, non-GMO "greens" and "reds" - which actually means many different colored fruits and vegetables, are the foods that are most associated with healthy aging. This is why I recommend juicing and supplemental green/red superfood powders that concentrate the best ingredients from many different vegetable and fruit sources.

The superfood powders are a way to end the decision of what healthy things to consume. With one scoop you can ingest the concentrated essences of many different foods for their curative effects. They gather the best ingredients from different sources and that large variety of easily absorbed micronutrients is a bonus for the tasks of cellular repair, including RNA and DNA repair, that is necessary for anti-aging. Together with fresh juicing, this is an excellent way to supply your body with beneficial micronutrients. This will help you look younger and feel younger.

Your diet is the entrance way to better health, and to live longer you don't have to become vegetarian but should bias your diet towards plants rather than meat consumption.

Chapter 6
Improve Your Home Environment

The ancients said that the life span of an individual has its own pattern, but meditation can increase your life span. The pattern of life includes all the activities of your life, therefore your longevity will strongly depend upon lifestyle factors.

As stated, the two basic principles for living longer include supplementation (augmentation or accumulation) and continuance (maintenance) strategies. To live longer you must focus on supplementing substances or essences that decline over time, and you must also focus on maintaining their levels and current healthy conditions so that they don't suffer from deterioration.

Putting it another way, pursuing longevity is a process of seeking to accumulate positive energies, influences and activities and avoiding their dissipation since this will result in loss.

At its core, the path of cultivating longevity involves cultivating your Qi, or life force energy. Cultivating your vital energy cannot be accomplished through a pill because it entails behavioral lifestyle changes such as the practice of meditation and the avoidance of harmful activities like smoking, taking drugs or eating the wrong foods. In a nutshell, you cultivate longevity by doing those behavioral things that will help your physical body and Qi rather than harm them.

What can you therefore do in your home in terms of better arranging your living environment to help with these efforts? Here are just a few of the important things that will help to maximize the healthy state of your home.

Clean Air

You cannot live without oxygen, so breathing clean air should be your number one priority in life. Your Qi (life force) and vitality are positively or negatively affected by the health of your respiratory system, your breathing patterns and the quality of the air you breath. Additionally, dirty air and oxygen deficiency promote and even cause disease over time – such as cancer, which cannot grow in a highly oxygenated cellular environment.

All sorts of healing therapies depend upon improving your blood circulation and delivering more oxygen to cells, but you cannot do that if the air you breathe is dirty or oxygen deficient.

Consider that all the breathing and pranayama exercises already mentioned are not only designed to affect the Qi of your body but to make your breathing processes more efficient so that you can get the maximum benefits from pure air and better oxygen uptake. But what if the air you breathe isn't pure due to pollutants?

Unfortunately, when there is smog and pollution in the air our health can suffer both from the decrease in oxygen levels and from the harmful effects of poisonous gases and particulates we inhale. Therefore, there are two types of airborne pollution that we need to particularly ban from our homes – (1) toxic gases and (2) particulate pollutants.

Let's talk about how to remove gases from our environment first, which means pollutants such as carpet odors, formaldehyde (from plywood outgassing), benzene fumes, furniture outgassing or paint fumes and the smell of household cleaners.

The two ways of removing gases from your home include air cleaners using activated carbon filters or ozone generators that chemically break down gases, vapors, odors in the air.

Carbon filters actually pull smells out of the air, and then neutralize the odors that pass through them. They chemically absorb gases and other impurities from any air that is pushed through the filters.

Ozone generators produce ozone that destroys odors in the air by oxidizing them. The problem with inexpensive ozone generators, however, is that they are usually poorly built such that they give off harmful gases in the form of nitrogen compounds along with the ozone. When using an ozone generator you should never smell the ozone. The trick to using a unit is to employ the highest setting you cannot smell and place the machine high up in a room so that as the ozone falls it spreads into the room as it is released. My favorite ozone generators are Aranizer units.

To eliminate particulate pollution in a room, which often helps asthma sufferers, there are several approaches possible:

(1) HEPA air filters,
(2) negative ion generators, and

(3) electrostatic precipitators (filters).

HEPA air filter devices suck particles out of the air and trap them with the filters, and are usually the most popular option. Aircare, Honeywell and many other firms manufacture high quality units. You'll have to check ratings sites (such as consumersearch.com or Consumer Reports) to determine which units are best as the standings are sure to change every so many years.

As to negative ion generators, they put a slight negative (ionic) charge on dust, pollen, and other pollutant particles and thereby cause them to precipitate out of the air onto non-living surfaces. This mimics the natural cleansing processes of nature found at the seashore, after storms, and near waterfalls. Despite this benefit, negative ions do not destroy odors. They only pull particles out of the air.

Negative ion generators are very helpful to individuals with breathing disorders as the ions they generate put charges on our lung's microfilaments to make them more efficient for breathing. Of the many manufacturers available I'm very fond of the Wein Products brand of ion generators because they often help asthma patients.

Electrostatic precipitators are air filters that remove fine air particles, like dust and smoke, by inducing an electrostatic charge as they are passing through metal collection plates. One advantage of these units is that they don't need expensive filters that must be replaced. However, a disadvantage is that they are messy to clean.

A final way to clean the air in your home is by using potted plants. NASA researcher Bill Wolverton studied the air cleaning capabilities of all sorts of houseplants and found special benefits from the Areca palm, Lady palm, Bamboo palm, Rubber plant, Dracaena (Janet Craig variety), English ivy, Dwarf date palm, Ficus alii, Boston fern, and Peace lily. Growing these plants inside your home would produce an extra boost to cleaner air.

Clean Water

Your body is composed of 70% water. You lose this water through perspiration and excretion, and therefore you need to replenish it on a daily basis. What is the best source? It is *not* distilled water, which is harmful to the body since it leaches your tissues of minerals.

Immortal Li drank fresh, clean spring water in the wilderness, but who else can do that? While there are many longevity characteristics attributed to special waters like this (Hunza water, glacial milk, Grander water, Willard water, microcluster water, alkaline water, etc.), the ordinary consumer has no regular access to these waters or cannot afford them.

Nobel Prize winner Dr. Henri Coanda studied five regions in the world where people lived exceptionally long lives and found that the only common factor which could explain their longevity was that they drank water from melted glaciers, which contained countless trace minerals. Once again, this emphasis on minerals for life extension is the same longevity principle found within Buddhism, Taoism, Ayurveda and the Siddha medical system once again. You need a steady supply of easily absorbed minerals in order to live longer.

Mountain waters and glacial waters are filled with minerals while distilled water is dead water devoid of everything, and actually robs your body of minerals if you drink it. Bottled water often contains harmful chemicals that have leached into it from the plastic container, and tap water usually contains fluoride, chlorine and heavy metals that must be filtered before drinking. Distilled, bottled and tap water therefore present potential problems if you want to drink clean, healthy water. Of these three, tap water is what you have in your home and what you usually depend upon the most, so to drink clean water you need to focus on filtering your tap water correctly.

In addition, because your skin is a sieve this means your body absorbs whatever lands on it. Thus you often absorb more chlorine into your body through a water shower than by drinking a glass of chlorinated tap water. You therefore need a solution for what you both drink *and* bathe in.

The chlorine in tap water is easy to remove using simple filters, but the secret key is to make sure that any filter contains a minimum of one pound of KDF (kinetic degradation fluxion), which is the magic filtering ingredient that removes chlorine, lead, mercury, iron and hydrogen sulfide from your water to purify it. Small faucet filters or shower filters are usually useless unless they contain a sufficient amount of KDF filtering material. If you want a good filter, make sure it has a sufficient NSF rating and a good amount of KDF.

Fluoride is more difficult to remove from water supplies except through distillation, reverse osmosis or activated alumina devices. Its removal requires far larger and more expensive filtering units for a home.

Basically, how much you can do for your water, such as even changing its alkalinity, depends upon how much you are willing to spend.

Reduce Your EMF Exposure

Electromagnetic radiation, microwaves, radio waves, and magnetic fields are now an ever increasing type of electronic pollution that is filling our homes and bathing our cells with harmful smog-like energies. We are constantly being bombarded by harmful EMF energies from Wifi devices, cell phones, microwave ovens, computers, our television and other electronic devices. Many people are becoming increasingly sensitive to all this EMF radiation. It is a growing problem attacking our health and longevity.

Here is why the increase in environmental EMF is a problem.

Living cells maintain an electrical charge across their membranes that is essential to their functioning, and which is sensitive to electromagnetic fields. Any radiation can disrupt this membrane potential, rearrange and damage cell molecules and therefore alter our metabolism in perverse ways.

EMFs also produce free radicals in cells which then accelerate the aging process. Furthermore, studies definitely link EMFs with tumors, leukemia, degenerative brain disease, breast cancer and other health conditions. Given all these negatives, what can you do to protect yourself since EMF pollution is increasing every year and now totally permeates most populated environments?

Here are just a few simple rules. Don't sleep under an electric blanket whose magnetic fields penetrate deeply into your body. Sit more than three meters away from the television and move away from microwave ovens when they are in use. Move electric clocks at least one meter from your head when you are sleeping. In general, reduce your radiation exposure of all types.

One of the biggest problems is cell phones since they generate a powerful burst of EMF energy when you dial another party, so at the minimum hold your cell phone at arm's length away from your ear when dialing and only bring it close to your ear after a connection has been established with the other party. To protect yourself, you can also find various cell phone protection devices at TooMuchEMF.com.

There are many solutions you can pursue to lower the harmful levels of EMF radiation in your home. I've spent many hours interviewing the oldest purveyor (and his staff) of EMF protective devices in the country to separate the scams from the few genuinely helpful devices and approaches that can protect you and your loved ones from all sorts of electrical, microwave and magnetic radiation.

You can find the result of those interviews (products that work at decreasing your risks due to EMF radiation) at TooMuchEMF.com.

Detoxification

Since the process of cultivating longevity involves meditation, and since meditation transforms the Qi and energy channels of your body within all your cellular tissues, the pursuit of longevity can actually be considered a process of transformation and purification. You are trying to purify your body of elements that shorten the life span, which is a transformation of its nature. This transformation involves the Jing, Qi and Shen of your nature – the physical body and its biochemical processes, the Qi life force of your body and the Qi channels within which it flows, and your mental spirit or Shen that needs to become more peaceful.

This process can also be termed "detoxification" because you must purge your body of accumulated cellular wastes, your Qi channel pathways must be cleared of blockages that obstruct the smooth flow of Qi within them, and your mind must be cleared of negative thoughts and habit energies that might harm you. Of particular importance are the methods used to clear your Qi channels of obstructions, which is why pranayama is recommended. The great Yoga sage Patanjali said that pranayama should be practiced daily so that "impurities are driven out of the body and purification occurs."

Whether through pranayama breathing practices or meditation or other techniques, impurities within your Qi channels are eliminated via expulsion, which is essentially a process of detoxification. We can also take herbs to help us discharge intestinal, liver and kidney wastes that build up in our tissues. My favorite consumer products along these lines are the Nature's Whole Body Program and Colon Cleanse together with Vitalzym. Most people who take these three products feel better and see their skin look younger after a few weeks of use.

The fact that aging cells collect intracellular and extracellular junk suggests that a good cellular house cleaning is in order if you are looking to avoid disease, look younger and live longer. Your body collects toxins and poisons in its organs and collective tissues, so a periodic detoxification (purification) routine would be most useful to any anti-aging efforts. Detoxification routines can certainly help cut down on your internal toxic load and reduce the potential causes behind various killer diseases such as cancer. They will also help you feel better, look better and live longer.

Detoxification is a complicated, multi-step process that can involve many substances and approaches. Here is a simple synopsis of the steps to take to detoxify your body.

First, stop adding to the problem of creating an even greater toxic load. Stop smoking, breathe cleaner air, drink cleaner water, stop exposing yourself to harmful chemicals, and change your diet so that you are eating clean foods and staying away from garbage junk food. With less poisons coming in, your body has a chance to catch up on cleansing your system of those already accumulated.

Second, start cleaning out any toxins that have already accumulated in your body, especially if you frequently experience constipation. Consider fasting, enemas or colonics for the intestines and various herbs and supplements used in detoxification routines for the liver, kidneys and connective tissues. *Detox Cleanse Your Body Quickly and Completely* can especially help in this regard because it teaches which supplements work best for cleaning every part of your body.

Third, "clean the pipes" within your body so that wastes can be more readily eliminated and excreted. This means improving the efficiency of your body's circulatory system and its channels of elimination.

For instance, the supplement nattokinase dissolves long-standing blood clots in veins and arteries, Detoxamin (a rectal suppository) chelates arterial walls to remove any unwanted mineral scaffolding, and the protocols of Linus Pauling and the Nobel Prize winning Doctors Robert Furchgott, Louis Ignarro and Ferid Murad can help to clean arteries and veins of excess plaque and cholesterol that coat their walls. PMCaox or Life Assure can do this as well if you take the product for about one year.

Fourth, increase blood circulation and oxygen exposure to your tissues via castor oil packs, deep tissue massage, chiropractic adjustments, yoga exercises or martial arts (stretching) and breathing exercises that help to open up Qi channels and circulatory routes via manual rather than chemical therapy.

Fifth, act to rebuild, strengthen, and nurture your health through good nutrition (a better diet) and targeted herbal, mineral and vitamin supplementation in order to activate, modulate and bolster the biochemistry responsible for healing and maintaining good health.

These are the few things you can do to improve your home environment to aid in your quest to stay healthy and live longer. By creating a healthy place to live that is free of pollutants you will maximize your chances for a healthier and longer life.

Chapter 7
Your Personal Steps
For Health And Longevity

Here is a quick summary of the steps you should take to maintain and improve your physical and inner energy body to look younger and live longer.

YOUR PHYSICAL BODY

1. Don't forget the obvious: avoid the accidents that normally kill people. Think safety first. In other words, don't do stupid things that can cause fatal injuries. If you want to live longer, take better care of yourself. Look both ways before crossing the street, use seatbelts, don't engage in dangerous sports, wear colorful clothes when riding a bike or hunting, don't travel on vacation to war zones, avoid exposing yourself to infectious diseases that might kill you and so forth. Use your brain to avoid what is dangerous because by avoiding fatal accidents you will certainly live longer.

2. Don't harm your body by adopting lifestyle factors that regularly kill people. Stop smoking and drinking to excess, and avoid drugs. Since a large number of people regularly die from cardiovascular disease or cancer, live life in such a way that your lifestyle thwarts these outcomes rather than makes them that much more likely.

If a job exposes you to dangerous chemicals, such as often happens in farming or chemical manufacturing, then take proper precautions to protect yourself so that you don't absorb deadly toxins. Take steps to avoid absorbing and accumulating toxic materials inside you and engage in regular detoxification regimes to get back to being toxin-free. Sickness is often due to biochemical imbalances caused by toxic accumulations, so the basic idea is to stop adding to the problem by taking preventative steps and clear out the problems that have accumulated through regular detoxification protocols.

3. Fast every now and then to help your body readjust itself. Intermittent fasting is healthy and helps you lose weight and look great.

4. Eat the right foods. Cut down on sugars and grains. Eat less, and primarily vegetarian. Eat a diet that is as much organic and non-GMO as possible. Only eat foods to which you are not sensitive or allergic. Add probiotic foods (such as kimchi, sauerkraut, natto, tempeh, pickles, kombucha, kefir or *real* yoghurt) to your diet. Consume as many colored foods as possible while avoiding the "whites" (wheat, bread, pasta, potatoes, rice) to a high degree since they spike your glucose levels. Consume good fats (cod liver oil, fish oil, olive oil, coconut oil, butter) instead of bad fats (corn oil, soybean oil, margarine, mayonnaise). Check out the Price-Pottenger Foundation (PPNF.org) for more information along these lines.

Eating the right foods is a supplementation and maintenance strategy, and the simplest way to supply yourself with the countless nutrients that will help with longevity efforts is to do fruit and vegetable juicing and consume a super green or super red powder on a daily basis whose many nutrient dense ingredients, in a powder form that makes them extremely easy to digest and absorb, takes away the problem of having to decide what individual foods or supplements to take. These nutrient-dense food powders help insure against insufficient minerals and healing nutrients in your diets. Rotate between different green/red brands as you finish any bottle so that you sequence through different formulas with different ingredients.

Remember to try raw fruit and vegetable juicing too despite the inconvenience. Juicing and super green/red powders will help to build, strengthen, and nurture your health. They will fulfill the requirement of eating supplemental foods, herbs, grasses and minerals that Shakyamuni Buddha and the Taoists recommended but without having to make decisions about selecting supplements. Even if you cannot follow these suggestions, follow this basic rule: eat healthy and don't eat crap.

Along these lines, don't forget to eat nucleotide-rich foods (which come from Breast milk, Sardines, Brewer's yeast, Anchovies, Mackerel, Lentils, most Beans, animal Liver, Oysters, Chlorella algae and Spirulina algae) since they readily supply the ingredients necessary for repairing RNA and DNA. Since Chlorella and Spirulina are in most green powders, you can get them in your diet through this particular avenue.

5. Maintain a clean living environment. Since your body is not only what you eat and drink but also what you absorb from the environment, make sure your house is a clean environment in terms of air quality, water quality, and EMF quality (see TooMuchEMF.com and CutCat.com).

6. Get regular chiropractic adjustments. This will improve your posture, fix any skeletal misalignments you might have developed, help your physical structure to stay in shape, and improve your blood circulation. The net result is that you will feel better and can often eliminate back pain without having to take medications, and the benefits will often be permanent. For postural help you might also pursue the Feldenkrais method, Aston patterning techniques and Egoscue.

Massage can also be helpful. Along these lines you might pursue Rolfing, Swedish massage, active-release technique (ART), advanced muscle integration therapy (AMIT), the Graston technique and other related modalities. Acupuncture and acupressure might also be helpful.

7. Keep your circulatory system cleansed of obstructions and open to blood flow. The circulatory system is the primary channel of nutrient supply and elimination in the body, and there are a wide variety of naturopathic approaches and nutritional supplements (nattokinase, Detoxamin EDTA, l-arginine, magnesium, gingko biloba, etc.) that can help dilate or clean the gunk out of veins and arteries that would normally impede excellent blood flow. Periodically use them.

8. Use vitamin-mineral-herbal nutritional supplements to correct any biochemical imbalances you already have and to provide helpful nutrients that might reverse conditions like diabetes, heart disease and cancer. The right diet and supplements can help turn back the biological clock. They can help prevent or alleviate health problems if they run in your family. As explained in my book *Move Forward,* you can use nutritional supplements to go against genetic predispositions and avoid or even reverse genetic tendencies that run in your family. You can defy your genes with the right nutritional supplements. Look to LEF.org for indications of which supplements might help a health condition or books like Jonathan Wright and Alan Gaby's *Nutritional Therapy in Medical Practice: Protocols and Supporting Information.*

9. Get plenty of sunshine. Light is also a nutrient just like food and is especially important for maintaining appropriate levels of vitamin D in your body. Most people are vitamin D deficient, which increases their susceptibility to cancer and other diseases. Being starved of light can also

lead to depression.

We have evolved under "full spectrum light" that includes UV energies, without which most plants won't bloom and fruits won't ripen, so spend some time each day in real sunshine. Sunshine is a food for your body that most doctors don't mention whose exposure satisfies one of the roads of supplemental practice (absorbing the energy of the sun) that Shakyamuni Buddha recommended for life extension.

10. Exercise regularly. It is a continuance-maintenance strategy that helps open up Qi channels and keep your body flexible. The results of various scientific studies definitely show that regular exercise reduces mortality and increases life expectancy, but it should be practiced in a gradual, prudent manner so you don't hurt yourself as you get older.

Since the "best exercise in the world" is useless if you don't practice it, the best exercise for you is the one which you will continue doing. Along these lines, look into gentle stretching exercises like yoga and Pilates, Z-health, and kettlebells. Kettlebells, in particular, are a great form of exercise that can help an overweight person become thin and a thin person gain muscles (weight).

Younger people should look into the benefits of using rebounders, power plates, and pogo sticks since they provide cardiovascular exercise, greatly stimulate your lymphatic system (one of your major detoxification systems), and are not likely to harm the joints of your body.

11. Detoxify regularly. Every year you should undergo some degree of herbal detoxification to rid your body of cellular wastes and organ toxins, especially in the channels of elimination that involve the intestines, liver and kidneys. Detoxification can help rid your body of acidic waste buildup that negatively impacts organs, which are worn down by toxins in our diet and environment.

The idea of purifying or transforming the physical body necessitates that you work towards cleaning out what is essentially a cesspool, so try to make sure that your channels of elimination are working properly and you have bowel movements every day.

In addition to the principles of the Blue Zones, these constitute the things you can do for your physical nature to look younger, feel better and live longer. Eat right, detoxify, ensure regular eliminations, exercise and stay socially active with a life purpose. If you do the right things you can live into the second half of your life free of all pain, discomfort and disease.

YOUR QI BODY

Since longevity is partly due to biochemistry and partly due to your life force, vital energy or Qi, you have to work on both factors for the best chances at life extension and looking younger. You must especially work on cultivating your vitality, which you can do through inner energy practices and meditation.

The biggest shock to people who want these goals is usually the fact that Qi exists and they have to work on accumulating their Qi life essence and opening up their Qi channels and on.

How do you open up your Qi channels?

1. The main route is through meditation practice, such as vipassana. See *The Little Book of Meditation, Twenty-Five Doors to Meditation, Visualization Power, Meditation Case Studies* and *Nyasa Yoga* for an excellent collection of easy but powerful meditation techniques.
2. Choose a form of martial arts (Tai chi, Akido, etc.), yoga practices or other stretching exercises (Pilates, Z-Health) that are suitable for you, and practice whatever you choose regularly. When combined with breath and movement, stretching can also help open up your Qi channels so that you look younger, feel better and live longer.
3. You can also use pranayama breathing practices, *disciplined* sexual intercourse, and mantra or even the energies of the environment as a supplemental force to help open up your energy channels all over your body. The best explanation of these techniques can be found in *Nyasa Yoga*.

The idea is to either use passive or active means to open up your energy channel pathways and when your Qi flows smoothly, without frictional loss due to internal challenges, you will build an independent life that can lend aid to the outer physical nature to help maintain it.

This is how to combine the Buddhist, Taoist, nutritional and western scientific road of principles you can and should use for super life extension.

Appendix 1
World Class Anti-Aging Supplements

Many times people seeking to use vitamin-mineral-herbal supplements to deal with health conditions and/or extend their longevity ask for opinions about the "best brands" or "best supplements" out there. Having surveyed countless nutritionists, manufacturers and doctors, I want to share some common conclusions from these interviews. The information does not constitute health advice but is simply intended to inform, so before using any supplements please check with your doctor who knows of your personal health conditions.

VITAMIN E

Probably the best vitamin E in the world (and only one I would ever recommend to those with health conditions that require vitamin E) is the A.C. Grace brand of vitamin E called "Unique E." The only product that the A.C. Grace company manufactures is triple-distilled, all natural vitamin E that is so effective it has been known to heal severe heart problems when the full dosage necessary is taken all at once for the day.

If any medical study shows that vitamin E "works" for a health condition, the results would probably be dramatically improved even more *if this particular brand of vitamin E was the one used in the trial.* If anyone in your family has cardiovascular problems or health conditions requiring vitamin E, this is the brand to consider.

VITAMIN C

Several studies suggest that supplementing with vitamin C at 2 grams/day probably adds four to six years to your life. The problem is which type of vitamin C is best. Mojo-C, with lipid metabolites, is a highly absorbable form of vitamin C that I personally use. Even so, I will change the type of vitamin C I use as superior new ones are developed and sold in the market. Freeda also makes a form of powdered, unbuffered vitamin C (called "Dull C") that has useful properties. Liv On Labs offers a lipospheric form of vitamin C. Different types of vitamin C are used for different purposes, but the ones used for strengthening arteries and veins should always be accompanied by bioflavonoids, which you can search for on the ingredients list.

B-VITAMINS

B-vitamins are commonly used for any nervous system related conditions such as stress or depression. In fact, the entire vitamin industry was started because people realized that the B-vitamin levels in our foods were plummeting because they start immediately degrading after food is picked on the farm, and too much time passes before the farmer's crop reaches our table. B-vitamins are very fragile to manufacture and last only hours in the body, meaning you should eat them twice or more per day as a vitamin supplement if you want to receive their maximum benefit. As with other vitamins, you should eat them with food – with the meal.

You can buy B-vitamins from many manufacturers, but an extremely strong consensus points to kosher manufacturer Freeda Vitamins as being at the very top of the list for the highest quality B-vitamin tablets and pills available. This is the preferred brand for pure B-vitamins due to their manufacturing process. Freeda's Ultra Freeda is also a simple multi-vitamin that you might consider as a daily supplement.

If I was interested in the metabolically active forms of B-vitamins such as methylcobalamin for vitamin B-12, pyridoxine HCl and Pyridoxyl-5-Phosphate for vitamin B-6, riboflavin HCl and riboflavin-5-phosphate for vitamin B-2, or even 5-MTHF for folate, many high quality manufacturers can supply a B-Complex supplement with the most biologically available forms of the B-vitamins. However, for the simple forms of vitamin B you can hardly go wrong with Freeda as a manufacturer.

MINERALS

For mineral supplementation, shilajit can be purchased from many different suppliers; it is difficult to determine the best brand although I generally like Jarrow as a low-cost, high quality supplier.

Trace minerals are important for the body, and I like liquid colloidal minerals since they supply minerals in an highly absorbable form, but once again it is difficult to determine a safe and reliable liquid colloidal mineral manufacturer since they often have too high an aluminum content. It you try a liquid colloidal mineral drink and then cannot sleep that night because of the extra energy then you know you definitely need trace mineral supplements in your diet. After a few days of this type of supplementation your body will get used to the extra energy boost.

For individual colloidal minerals such as gold, silver, copper and zinc, PurestColloids makes the smallest colloidal minerals on the planet due to a unique manufacturing process not employed elsewhere in the world. Its liquid colloidal minerals have extremely tiny molecular sizes and thus provide extremely high therapeutic benefit. Available in small bottles or gallon jugs, these are the ones preferred for therapeutic applications.

Other notable mineral brands include Goldstake Minerals and Trace Mineral Research. Kelp tablets are also a way to ingest more minerals from sea vegetable sources.

HEAVY METALS

Countless products are available to help in eliminating heavy metals from the body. Among the best heavy metal detoxifiers are Heavy Metal Nan Detox (from PrLabs) and Modifilan algae capsules. Modifilan also has anti-cancer properties.

SELENIUM

A superior form of selenium is available as Phytosel, which is natural selenium from hydroponically grown mustard greens. This plant-based selenium seems to be much better absorbed than other forms of selenium.

JOINT PAIN

Many people develop joint pain as they get older and try supplement after supplement seeking a solution to their discomfort. They usually run through glucosamine sulfate, chondroitin sulfate, MSM and other products without obtaining relief. For joint pain they might try the very inexpensive Neocell Collagen Type 2 or Jarrow Type 2 Collagen, made of hydrolyzed chicken sternal cartilage, that has been known to stop pain completely or reduce it dramatically in just days. Neocell Collagen 1 & 3 also works. It's an inexpensive "miracle" product for knee pain and other joint pain issues that might help you avoid surgery.

FISH OIL

I prefer the Pharmax brand of fish oil capsules, which is the brand the India government has selected to use after carefully studying all the products on the market. This is a brand that gets results whereas cheap fish oil products, purchased at bargain prices, usually do nothing for you because of the low quality. If you are going to buy fish oil, buy the best and get the promised health results rather than cheap stuff that delivers nothing at all.

For regular vegetable oils, the Omega brand is one of the few manufacturers that cold presses the oils in darkened rooms to avoid lipid oxidation where the oils spoil before they are even sold. Another product that impresses me is micro-milled lecithin granules found in individually sealed packets so as to also prevent oxidation and spoilage. This type of product, made from non-GMO soybeans (the only source I found is from Russia), would be excellent for building the brain, especially of growing kids, because of its high fat content. Expensive, it is also a wonderful supplement for the skin.

DETOX PROTOCOLS

To make it simple, the detoxification regime I use on a yearly basis involves three products. Nature's Pure Body Whole Body Program plus Colon Program, and Vitalzym. These products alone will start making you look and feel younger. In *Detox Cleanse Your Body Quickly and Completely* I describe how to detox every part of your body.

PARASITES

There are many parasite products in the marketplace which depend on herbal ingredients like Black Walnut, Wormwood, Goldenseal, Oregon Grape Root or cloves. PC 123 (from BCN4Life.com) is one of the best. It was formulated to be safe enough to use 365 days per year and despite a gentle nature seems to work on almost everything – yeast, amoebas, protozoa, worms and everything that causes diarrhea. It is like a broad spectrum anti-microbial, but it doesn't seem to disturb good gut flora and has ingredients that also strengthen the immune function of the gut as it is being used.

Because I travel internationally and eat all sorts of strange foods, every few years I do a parasite detox by using two bottles of this product. I add it to the Nature's Pure Body Whole Body Program plus Colon Program and Vitalzym protocol.

MUSHROOMS

Mushroom Science / JHS Natural Products is one of the world's best manufacturers of mushroom supplements and has an excellent immune building supplement called Immune Builder. Hyperimmune egg powder (such i26) is another immune building product that can be helpful. Another notable immune builder product is 4Life Transfer Factor Plus. Madre Labs also makes an immune powder (Immune Punch) that you can readily add to a green powder superfood. In this case, Immune Punch contains Epicor (dried yeast complex), AHCC, and a variety of immune enhancing mushroom extracts. While beneficial, the problem with immune builders of all types is that they usually take a few months to kick in.

ENERGY

Cardiovascular patients, and in particular those taking statin drugs, often have less energy and are told to take CoQ10. The Jarrow brand of Coenzyme Q10 (QH + PQQ or Q-absorb) is my preferred brand because the ubiquinol comes directly from the Japanese manufacturer. This form of ubiquinol CoQ10 seems to be more readily absorbed than many other types of CoQ10. It actually works at making people feel better and changing their blood markers. Unfortunately, many supplement manufacturers use CoQ10 supplied from low quality Chinese producers whose product quality just doesn't seem to produce the same health benefits.

Normally I would prefer Bio-Quinon Pharma Nord CoQ10 since it is an excellent European manufacturer that I believe is the best in the marketplace, but unfortunately its product is not readily available in the U.S. market. Sometimes you can find it available on amazon.com.

All heart conditions are usually signs of energy deficiency and the primary intervention would be CoQ10 (as well as magnesium, such as AOR's CardioMag). Even detox efforts are better accomplished when you take CoQ10 as well.

CLEAN ARTERIES

Speaking of cardiovascular problems, nattokinase is a blood clot-busting miracle supplement that often lowers your blood pressure permanently. Check out the Allergy Research/Nutricology brand (pearl capsules preferred) for a reliable nattokinase product that also comes directly from a high quality Japanese manufacturer. Pharmaceutical drugs offer a better, quicker and more predictable solution to blood clotting issues, but for prevention purposes this is a supplement your doctor should look into.

As to cleaning your arteries of accumulated cholesterol, the many approaches you can try (such as stripping your arteries clean through a combination of vitamin K, vitamin C, vitamin E and PhosChol supplementation) often work, but can lead to buildups again after the supplementation protocol stops. Detoxamin is a form of at-home chelation therapy, but the government may outlaw the supplement because of the obvious benefits.

The Nobel Prize winning work of Ignarro, Furchgott and Murat suggests that arginine and other amino acids may increase nitrous oxide in the arteries and strip them clean, but it seems to either work for you or your problem gets worse, suggesting there may be something in an individual that is required for best results along these lines. Even if this works, if you stop using this approach then the problem often comes back.

Evidence also suggests that arterial plaque, hypertension, and cancer disappear in populations when phytosterols are once again sufficiently found in the diet. Unfortunately, they have been removed since the time the modern food industry started taking fatty acids and other substances out of foods to prevent them from rotting between the time they leave the farm and arrive at your table.

Phytosterols are found primarily in vegetable sources, and for longevity and good health you should have a preference towards local foods and a fresh organic vegetable-based diet. An approach like CoQ10 with vitamin K (K1 and K2) and high levels of phytosterols (in products like PMCaox or Life Assure) along with niacin (250 mg/day – Freeda's time-release) can slowly strip arterial plaques clean starting in six to seven months to two years.

SUGAR CONTROL

There are many approaches to sugar control, which is the natural result of a calorie restriction diet and a key principle to any efforts at life extension and anti-aging.

Under the guidance of a professional, products such as AOR's beneGene (3-carboxy-3-oxopropanoic) can be used for excellent blood sugar regulation. This is the type of product that resets your cellular genetic switches to when you were about twenty-three years old. A combination of Berberine (Thorne Research) and Cinnamon (Pure Encapsulations) is another way to help dramatically lower blood sugar levels.

Many other approaches are possible depending on your conditions. Powerful products containing adaptogens and special co-factors such as Life Assure (BCN Formulas) and PMCaox supply powerful phytosterols that help restore cellular elasticity so that insulin can get into cells. Individuals who first undertake a systematic cleanse – such as by using Nature's Pure Body product, Vitalzym and PC 123 – and then work at a better diet, sugar control and restoring cellular membrane elasticity have a good chance at reversing many health problems.

EMF PRODUCTS

TooMuchEMF.com contains a short list of anti-radiation, anti-microwave, anti-dirty electricity and anti-EMF pollution devices that actually work for your office and home. If you have a cell phone, check it out to keep abreast of the latest protections available that will help protect you from getting a brain tumor due to too much careless cell phone usage. Simple things can protect you. Since silver is likely to increase in price over the years, any silver-based products (clothing or bed canopies) that protect your from EMF might be a good investment sooner rather than later.

A SIMPLE ANTI-AGING REGIME

When people me ask me what fewest products I would personally use for the most powerful anti-aging longevity regime I tell them to ponder the following but check with their doctor for advice.

Every year I do something for my body in terms of detoxification, and so should you. I personally use at least one bottle of **Nature's Pure Body Whole Body Program** and **Nature's Pure Body Colon Program** once per year, along with a bottle of **Vitalzym**. This cleans the body of many accumulated toxins and you can immediately see the result by the fact your skin becomes noticeably lighter as toxins are eliminated from connective tissues. Of course more complicated protocols are available, but this is the simplest protocol that seems the most helpful for people.

The Nature's Pure Body products help cleansing at the cellular level, which frees up the CoQ10 inside cells so that they don't have to be preoccupied with removing cellular wastes. With the extra CoQ10 your cells can then devote their maximal energies to DNA/RNA repair mechanisms. For extra CoQ10 I take **Jarrow's QH + PQQ**, which is CoQ10 plus PQQ (pyrroloquinoline quinone), a micronutrient the ancients didn't know about that helps stimulate the formation of new mitochondria in our cells. That's a good thing because having extra mitochondria around will help boost your energy and fight illness. You only need about 15/mg PQQ per day. Whenever I can buy it I take **Bio-Quinon Pharma Nord CoQ10** instead.

Because my diet isn't always what it should be, I would like to be juicing fruits and vegetables but this isn't always possible. Therefore I daily consume a mixture of **green powders** (phytonutrient-rich plant powders such as Boku Superfoods powder, Rejuvenate Plus, Green Vibrance, Madre Labs Midori Greens, Vitamineral Green, etc.) and **red powders** (such as Nutricology's ProBerry-Amla) to supply my body with as many different micronutrients as possible that can be used to help support and repair my cells. As a result of this supplementation, I don't need to go through any complicated daily decision process on extra supplements to take. I'm getting my phytochemicals through my foods, through juicing and through these nutrient-rich powders.

Combination products like Paradise Herbs ORAC-Energy Greens and Living Fuel Superberry Ultimate are superfoods that combine herbs together with other vegetables, minerals, vitamins and protein sources for one stop nutritional shopping. To cover your nutritional bases, you basically just choose several of these types of product and switch between them on a daily basis. The juicing of freshly picked, raw vegetables and fruits is a better choice, but since that is inconvenient or costly for most people I mention this solution. These powders can and should be added to juicing.

I use Robert Bard's **PMCaox** to obtain antioxidants, adaptogens an phytosterols that aren't in my diet while a cheaper version with fewer ingredients is **Life Assure** from BCN Formulas. I also take the **BCM-95** full spectrum Curcumin to help manage blood sugar levels, reset genetic switches and help protect against cancer.

The reason most people don't get well by taking supplements is because they are lacking a Core Nutritional Supplementation program. This is key. That core program would include **CoQ10 (Bio-Quinon or Jarrow) + Phytosterols (PMCaox or Life Assure) + Curcumin (BCM-95) + Antioxidants (Freeda or Thorne vitamins).**

B-vitamins degrade over time, so even though superfoods amply supply micronutrients and herbs to help repair RNA/DNA and support other biochemical processes, you might want to supply your body with a good B-vitamin on a daily basis, such as from a company like Freeda. A vitamin-mineral supplement should always be consumed with meals because that will ensure the best absorption.

For multi-vitamins I like the Freeda, Thorne and Super Nutrition brands. For general supplements I prefer the AOR, Jarrow, and Thorne brands. For minerals I use a **shilajit** supplement.

Basically the formula for health and anti-aging is **Food** [Organic Juicing + Red/Greens + Nucleotide-rich foods] + **Herbs** [Curcumin & Resveratrol & Carotenoids & Phytosterols] + **Vitamins & Minerals & Biochemical Co-factors** [Shilajit + CoQ10 & PQQ + B-vitamins] = greater health and longevity.

As you can see, this approach combines the Taoist and Buddhist regimes along with modern scientific insights. I believe it provides the best chances for super health and longevity purposes. It addresses the modern scientific and nutritional lines of thinking concerning the many causative theories of aging, and also follows the supplementation and maintenance thoughts of the ancient Taoists and Buddhists who were masters of longevity.

If you add the practice of meditation and stretching to this list, and also watch your diet, then this is a simple and pretty complete approach to health and longevity.

If the issue was nutritionally preparing children to have the best bodies for life (or preparing them for super performance in sports or chosen activities such as spiritual cultivation), I would heavily rely on the nutritional advice of the Price Pottenger Foundation.

I would also make sure that youngsters had ready access to GMO-free organic fruits and vegetables, free range meats, fresh vegetable and fruit juicing drinks, red powders and green powder drinks, shilajit for minerals, clean vegetable oils and micro-milled lecithin (for the brain and connective tissues), cod liver oil in milk (for beautiful skin) and bone broth soups (to help build strong joints). Children might also take a daily vitamin supplement and of course should avoid food sensitivities and allergenic foods.

By flooding the body with nutrients in the early growth years – making countless nutrients readily available so that the body can pick and choose what it needs – you will give young bodies the greatest chance to avoid vitamin-mineral and nutrient deficiencies and grow such that they express their maximum genetic potential.

Appendix 2
Optimal Blood Test Reference Ranges

Most people don't know that there are many tools available that nutritionists, physicians, naturopaths and you can use to help make better choices in choosing vitamin-mineral supplements for health and anti-aging efforts.

For instance, some of the more thorough and scientifically researched nutritional protocol books include:

- Jonathan Wright and Alan Gaby's *Nutritional Therapy in Medical Practice: Protocols and Supporting Information*
- Melvyn Werbach and Jeffrey Moss's *Textbook of Nutritional Medicine*
- The Life Extension Foundation's *Disease Prevention and Treatment*.

Many times the early indications that your internal biochemistry is somehow imbalanced can be spotted in your blood work; and then a subclinical health problem can be easily restored to normal through the correct approach of vitamin-mineral supplements. However, you need to use "optimal reference ranges" rather than standard reference ranges for the blood markers in order to spot these imbalances early, which can also help shed light on hard-to-diagnose conditions.

Where can you get optimal reference ranges for blood tests that you can use to compare with your own results?

These ranges can trace their origins to those published and copyrighted by Harry Eidinier, Jr., Ph.D. in *Balancing Body Chemistry*, and you can find similar ranges in the works of biochemist and physician Nick Abrishamian, Dr. Jack Tipps, Dr. R. M. Cessna, and others. They are worth their weight in gold to those with hard to diagnose health problems.

For your reference in trying to determine how to nutritionally intervene for a health condition, here are the optimal ranges most commonly reported from their work and within *Blood Chemistry and CBC Analysis* (Bear Mountain Publishing, Jacksonville: Oregon, 2002, p. 280), by Dick Weatherby and Scott Ferguson, which I encourage people to purchase for their home use:

Glucose	80-100
HgB A1C	4.1-5.7%
BUN	10-16
Creatinine	0.8-1.1
Sodium	135-142

Potassium	4.0-4.5
Chloride	100-106
CO2	25-30
Anion Gap	7-12
Uric Acid	3.5-5.9 male; 3.0-5.5 female
Total Protein	6.9-7.4
Albumin	4.0-5.0
Calcium	9.2-10.0
Phosphorus	3.0-4.0
Gastrin	45-90
Alk Phosphatase	70-100
SGOT (AST)	10-30
SGPT (ALT)	10-30
LDH	140-200
Total Bilirubin	0.1-1.2 (>2.6)
Direct Bilirubin	0-0.2 (>0.8)
Indirect Bilirubin	0.1-1.0 (>1.8)
GGTP	10-30
CPK	30-180
Globulin	2.4-2.8
Alpha 1 Globulin	0.2-.3
Alpha 2 Globulin	0.6-.9
Beta Globulin	0.7-1.0
Gamma Globulin	1.0-1.5
A/G Ratio	1.4-2.1
Bun/Creatinine	10-16
Cholesterol	150-220
Triglycerides	70-110
LDL	<120
HDL	>55
Chol/HDL	<4
Total Iron	50-100
Ferritin	33-26 males; 10-122 female
TIBC	250-350
TSH	2.0-4.4
T-3 Uptake	27-37
T-3	100-230
T-4 Thyroxine	6-12
WBC	5.0-7.5
RBC	4.2-4.9 male; 3.9-4.5 female
Reticulocytes	0.5-1
Hemoglobin	14-15 male; 13.5-14.5 female
Hematocrit	40-48 male; 37-44 female

MCV	82-89.9
MCH	28-31.9
MCHC	32-35
Platelets	150,000-385,000
RDW	<13
Neutrophils	40-60%
Lymphocytes	24-44%
Monocytes	0-7%
Eosinophils	0-3%
Basophils	0-1%

ABOUT THE AUTHOR

Bill Bodri is the author of several business, investing, health and self-help books including:

- *Quick, Fast, Done: Simple Time Management Secrets from Some of History's Greatest Leaders*
- *How to Create a Million Dollar Unique Selling Proposition*
- *Breakthrough Strategies of Wall Street Traders: 17 Remarkable Traders Reveal Their Top Performing Investment Strategies*
- *Super Investing: 5 Proven Methods for Beating the Market and Retiring Rich*
- *High Yield Investments, Hard Assets and Asset Protection Strategies*
- *Super Cancer Fighters*
- *The Little Book of Meditation*
- *Meditation Case Studies*
- *Nyasa Yoga*
- *Visualization Power*
- *Detox Cleanse Your Body Quickly and Completely*

If you liked this book you will most probably find *Detox Cleanse Your Body Quickly and Completely* of great interest since it teaches you how to detox your body of toxic substances that build up within the body over time. *Nyasa Yoga* would be of particular interest to those who wish to pursue meditation and inner energy work techniques to cultivate their Qi and energy channels.

The author can be contacted for interviews or speeches through wbodri@gmail.com.

29808566R00055

Made in the USA
San Bernardino, CA
18 March 2019